20 Months to a Champion Physique
Beginner Programs - Months 1 through 6

Written and Published by Bill Pearl
Edited by George and Tuesday Coates
Layout and Illustrations by Richard R. Thornley Jr.

Bill Pearl
P.O. Box 1080
Phoenix, Oregon 97535
Email: support@billpearl.com
Website: www.billpearl.com

ISBN-13: 978-1-938855-12-2

Notice of Rights

Medical Disclaimer - See Your Doctor

Please get a physical before starting any of the programs in this book, especially if you are overweight, have not exercised for a while, have had any health problems or if there is any history of health problems. We also recommend that you then visit your doctor on a regular basis while training and report any problems to your doctor.

Should any exercises in these routines be uncomfortable or dangerous to do because of some sort of physical impairment you have, please substitute another exercise for the same body part which will not aggravate the condition. There is a tremendous variety of exercises available for any body part, as you know if you have seen or read my book, *Keys to the Inner Universe*, so there's absolutely no reason to be doing some particular exercise that aggravates a back problem, a weak knee or whatever condition you may have simply because you see it in a workout routine somebody put together.

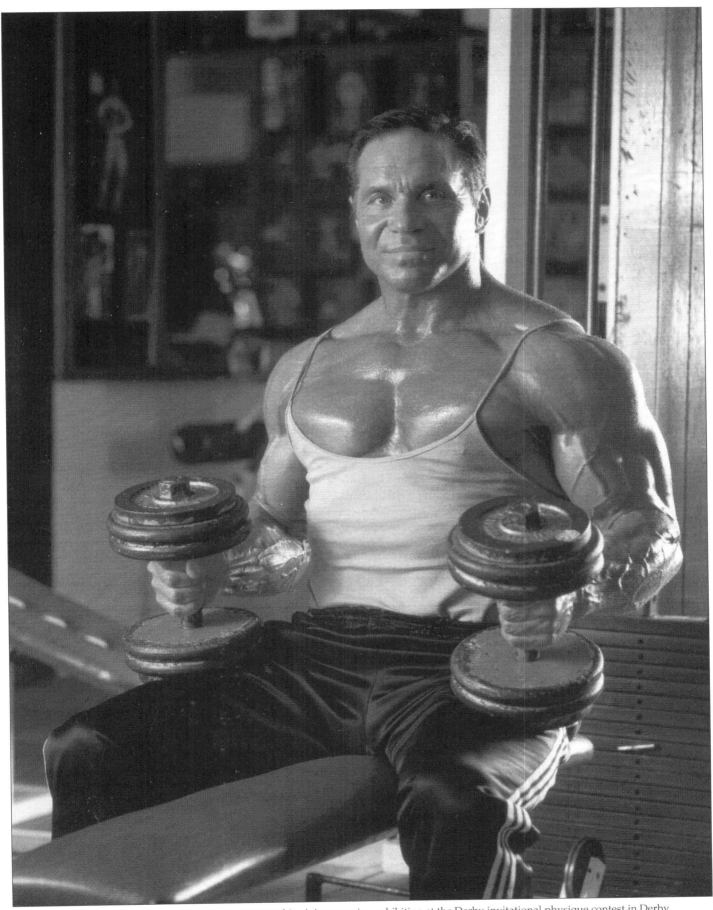

This photo was taken on Bill's 55th birthday just prior to his giving a posing exhibition at the Derby invitational physique contest in Derby, England. Photo by Chris Lund.

Table of Contents

Chapter 1

Do Not Train to Failure

People ask me why I don't believe in training to failure at a time when the popular notion in bodybuilding is that the only way to make maximum progress is to always go for that last impossible rep (in other words, train to failure). I tell them the answer is quite simple: If you do a workout of, say, nine exercises, three sets per exercise, and in each set you go to failure, which means you couldn't complete the last rep, what you have done in these 27 sets is trained yourself to fail 27 times! That doesn't sound like success in my book.

My approach to training has always been to push yourself in your workouts, but do not train to failure! The last rep should be difficult, but not impossible or unachievable. And I've always been a great believer that you should leave the gym each day feeling like you had a great workout but you've still got a little bit left in the gas tank, so to speak. Because if you don't leave the gym with the feeling of having something in reserve, you will sooner or later reach a point where your training begins to seem so hellish and burdensome, you will either start missing workouts or stop training altogether. And then where is your progress?

So speaking from experience, I urge you: Train hard, yes, but not to failure. Complete what you start -- and that means every rep. I believe that this approach will not only ensure that you'll stay with your training program year after year (obviously training longevity is a very important aspect of all of this) but you'll also make the greatest progress. Why? Because you'll be training yourself for success in each and every rep, set and workout. Your training will be a positive rather than negative experience. And you'll be much more likely to keep your enthusiasm high and to avoid injury, overtraining and mental burnout.

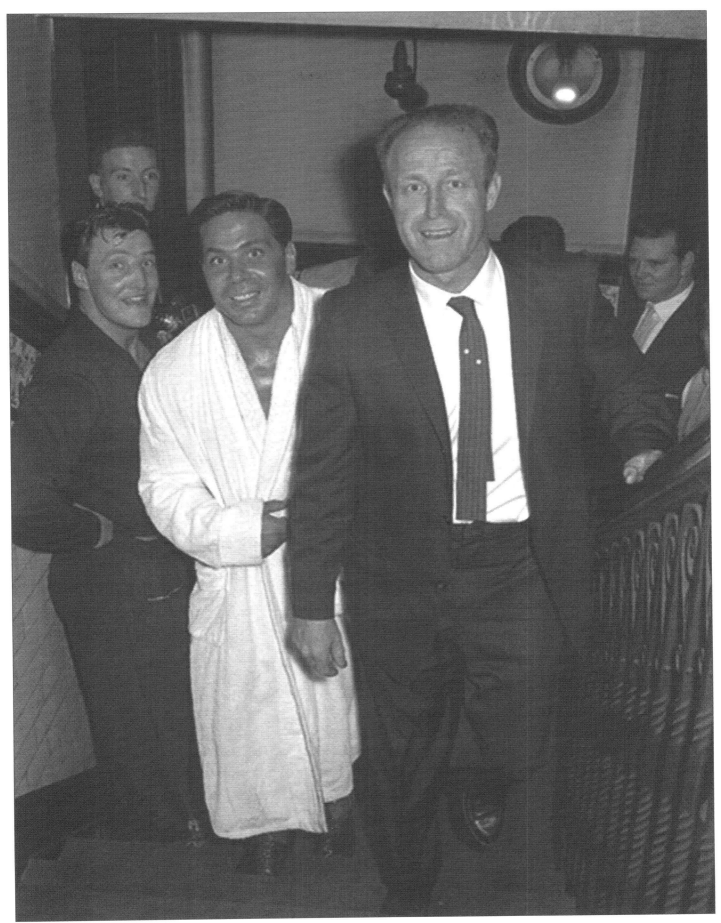

Leo Stern escorting Bill Pearl to the stage of the 1961 Mr. Universe competition which Bill won.

Chapter 2

Month One

Exercise	
1. Thigh Extension on Leg Extension Machine	3 sets of 12 reps
2. Medium Grip Barbell Bench Press	3 sets of 12 reps
3. Standing Dumbbell Upright Rowing	3 sets of 12 reps
4. Close Grip Straight Arm Lat Pulldown	3 sets of 12 reps
5. Straight Arm Dumbbell Pullover	3 sets of 12 reps
6. Standing Dumbbell Triceps Curl	3 sets of 12 reps
7. Standing Medium Grip Barbell Curl	3 sets of 12 reps
8. Heel High Sit-Up	3 sets of 10-30 reps
9. Flat Bench Leg Pull-In	3 sets of 10-30 reps

Congratulations! You are about to embark on a progressive weight training program which will take you from the Beginner to the Intermediate and on up to the Advanced level in the next 20 months. I have always been a great believer in incorporating a lot of variety into my training regimen. Consequently, in this 20-month program, we will change the exercises and the training routine every month, In addition, we will also vary the order in which the various body parts are trained.

One result of all this variety, I think you will find, is that your training will be much more interesting and your bodybuilding progress much greater. Why? Because you will be keeping your training fresh from month to month, and you will be hitting the muscles from so many angles. An additional benefit of all this, of course, is that by the end of the 20 months, you will be familiar with such a large number of weight training exercises, you will really be an expert on how to work any muscle from any angle to produce the desired results.

As you proceed through this program, you will have the option of doing the workouts as we've described them month to month -- six months for the Beginner level, six for the Intermediate level, and eight for the Advanced level. If, however, you wish to take longer to go from one level to the next, you can stay on a particular routine longer -- e.g., six weeks or two months -- which would ultimately expand this into a 30- or 40-month program. Generally speaking, however, I recommend that you change your exercises at least every six weeks; otherwise, your muscles start adapting to the particular movement and your progress slows.

You also have the option of going to a certain level of difficulty in this program and electing not to train any harder. For example, you may want to work up to the intensity of Month 12, the end of the Intermediate level, and no further. It's totally up to you. What we are giving you here is a tried and tested program which is guaranteed to give you exciting results if you follow it and really apply yourself. But you are the one doing the work, you know what you want, how far you seek to go with your bodybuilding, how much time, energy and dedication you have to apply to this, etc. So ultimately you are the one who has to decide exactly what you want to do and accomplish. My role is simply to provide you with some direction and whatever expertise I've been able to acquire in the 50 plus years I've been a bodybuilder.

Should any exercises in these routines be uncomfortable or dangerous to do because of some sort of physical impairment you have, please substitute another exercise for the same body part which will not aggravate the condition. There is a tremendous variety of exercises available for any body part, as you know if you have seen or read my book, Keys to the Inner Universe, so there's absolutely no reason to be doing some particular exercise that aggravates a back problem, a weak knee or whatever condition you may have simply because you see it in a workout routine somebody put together.

If you are a fairly experienced or even advanced bodybuilder accustomed to much high training loads than we have prescribed in the initial workouts here, don't worry! My suggestion would be: Take a break from the higher workload you've been doing, start back in at this lower level, and progressively build back up. Believe me, soon enough in this program the workload will increase to a level which you will find more than challenging -- regardless of your training background.

One last note, in this initial routine and all the others during the first 10 months, you will train your entire body in each workout. But starting with Month 11, which will be the latter part of the Intermediate phase, we'll switch to a split routine in which you will train half your body in one workout, the other half in the next one.

Training Suggestions for Month 1

- For best results, do this routine three times a week -- Monday, Wednesday and Friday, or Tuesday, Thursday and Saturday, Use the off days for rest and recuperation, which your body will need, particularly if you're new to weight training.
- Your weekly progression should be as follows:
  - Week 1: one set and minimum reps (i.e., the suggested number of reps unless there is a range).
  - Week 2: The suggested sets and medium reps (where a range is indicated).
  - Week 3 and 4: Full sets and reps.
- In the case of the two abdominal exercises included in this routine, start each exercise with the minimum number of reps and add a few reps at each workout until you reach the maximum number.
- How much weight should you use in these various exercises? Use as much weight as is comfortable for the reps indicated. The last rep should feel difficult, but should NOT be an all-out effort.
- As you continue training and your strength improves, the poundages you've been using will feel easy. Whenever you reach that point, increase the poundage until the last rep is difficult again. Always keep accurate records of your exercises, sets and reps from workout to workout, week to week, month to month. This will enable you, among other things, to keep track of your progress from one poundage to the next rather than making the whole process haphazard. Don't get caught up in always trying to top yourself from workout to workout. Remember what we said earlier: The last rep should feel difficult but should not be an all-out effort.
- Concentrate on correct form when doing each exercise.
- Inhale as you lower the weight and exhale forcefully on the exertion phase of the movement.
- Rest for 30 seconds to two minutes between sets. If you feel pain or need any kind of help during your workout, check with a trainer (if one is available).
- Of course, you should always consult with a physician before undertaking a training program to ensure that you have no health problems which could make training dangerous for you.

THIGH EXTENSION ON LEG EXTENSION MACHINE

Muscle Group: Lower thighs

Degree of Difficulty: Intermediate

Sit at the end of a leg extension machine placing the top part of your ankles and feet under the lower foot pads. Back up far enough on the seat to keep the end of the seat against the rear of your knees. Hold on to the seat with both hands just behind your buttocks. Point your toes slightly downward. Inhale and raise the weight stack until your legs are parallel with the floor. Return to starting position and exhale. Keep your upper body in a fixed position during the exercise.

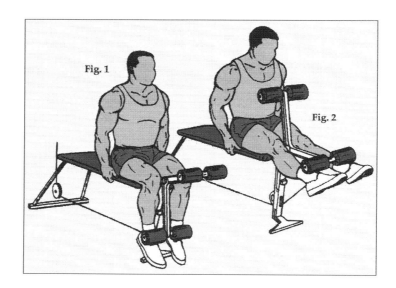

Sets/Reps: 3 sets of 12 reps

Date	Set One		Set Two		Set Three	
	Reps	Weight	Reps	Weight	Reps	Weight

Muscle Group: Outer pectorals

Degree of Difficulty: Intermediate

Lie in a supine position on a flat bench with your legs positioned at the sides of the bench and your feet flat on the floor. Using a hand grip that is about six inches wider than your shoulder width, bring the barbell to arm's length above the chest but in line with the shoulders. Lower the barbell to a position on the chest that is about an inch below the nipples of the pectorals. Note from figure 1 that the elbows are back and the chest is held high. Inhale as the barbell is lowered to the chest and exhale as you push the barbell back to arm's length. Do not relax and drop the weight on the chest but lower it with complete control making a definite pause at the chest before pressing it back to starting position. Keep the head on the bench and do not arch the back too sharply as to raise your hips off the bench.

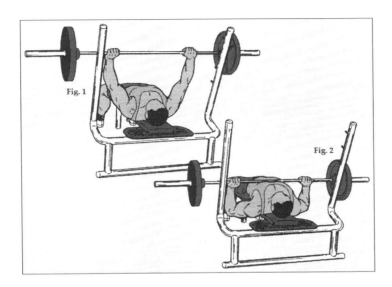

Sets/Reps: 3 sets of 12 reps

Date	Set One		Set Two		Set Three	
	Reps	Weight	Reps	Weight	Reps	Weight

Muscle Group: Front deltoids and trapezius

Degree of Difficulty: Intermediate

Use a dumbbell in each hand held at arm's length against your upper thighs. You should keep the dumbbells about ten inches apart during the exercise and have your thumbs facing each other. Inhale and pull the dumbbells straight up until they are nearly even with your chin. You must keep the elbows out to the sides and in the top position the elbows will be nearly as high as your ears. Keep the weights in close to the body and pause momentarily at the top. Concentrate as you lower the dumbbells to the starting position. Inhale up and exhale down.

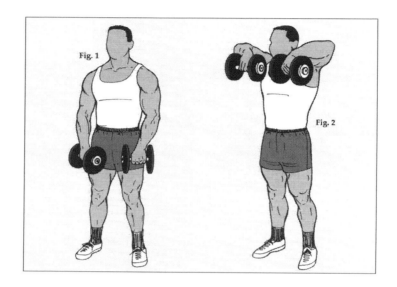

Sets/Reps: 3 sets of 12 reps

Date	Set One		Set Two		Set Three	
	Reps	Weight	Reps	Weight	Reps	Weight

Muscle Group: Lats

Degree of Difficulty: Intermediate

Place your hands on a lat machine bar about eight inches apart. Step back away from the lat machine until you are supporting the weight stack with your arms while they are extended in front of you about to the height of your head. Inhale and pull the bar straight down keeping your arms locked until the bar touches the top of your thighs. Return to starting position and exhale.

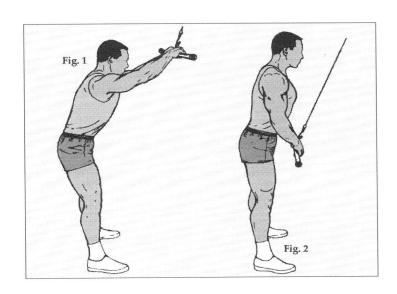

Sets/Reps: 3 sets of 12 reps

Date	Set One		Set Two		Set Three	
	Reps	Weight	Reps	Weight	Reps	Weight

STRAIGHT ARM DUMBBELL PULLOVER

Muscle Group: Pectorals and rib cage

Degree of Difficulty: Intermediate

Lie supine on a flat bench with your head as close to the end of the bench as possible. Place your hands flat against the inside plate of a dumbbell. With the dumbbell held at arm's length above the chest, take a deep breath and lower the dumbbell in a semicircular motion over the chest and head to a position behind your head that brings no discomfort to the shoulder area. From this position, return the dumbbell to starting position, still keeping the elbows in a locked position. Exhale as you reach the starting position. Keep the head down, your chest held high, breathe deeply and do not raise your hips off the bench.

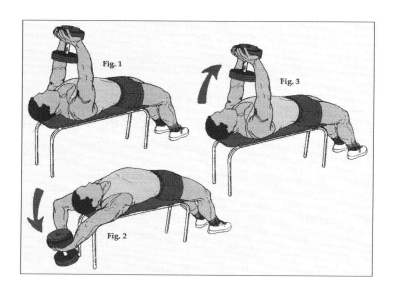

Sets/Reps: 3 sets of 12 reps

Date	Set One		Set Two		Set Three	
	Reps	Weight	Reps	Weight	Reps	Weight

Muscle Group: Triceps
Degree of Difficulty: Difficult

Grasp one dumbbell with both hands and raise it overhead to arm's length, vertical with the floor. As you are raising the dumbbell rotate your hands up and over until the top plates are resting in the palms of your hands while your thumbs remain around the handle. Stand erect with your back straight, head up and feet about sixteen inches apart. Keep your upper arms in close to the sides of your head during the exercise. Inhale and lower the dumbbell behind your head in a semicircular motion until your forearms and biceps touch. Return the weight to starting position using a similar path and exhale.

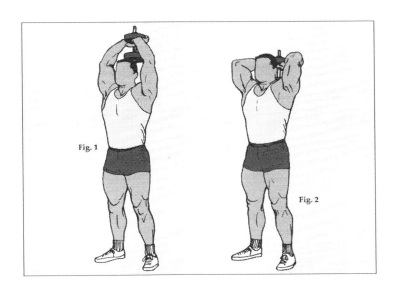

Sets/Reps: 3 sets of 12 reps

Date	Set One		Set Two		Set Three	
	Reps	Weight	Reps	Weight	Reps	Weight

Muscle Group: Biceps

Degree of Difficulty: Intermediate

Hold a barbell with both hands using a palms-up grip about eighteen inches apart. Stand erect with your feet about sixteen inches apart. With the barbell at arm's length against your upper thighs, inhale and curl the bar up to the height of your shoulders keeping your back straight, legs and hips locked out. As you are lowering the bar back to starting position, do so in a controlled manner causing the biceps to resist the weight as much as possible. Exhale as you return to starting position.

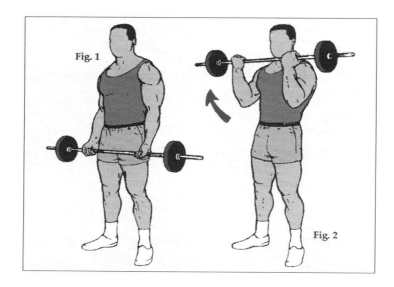

Sets/Reps: 3 sets of 12 reps

Date	Set One		Set Two		Set Three	
	Reps	Weight	Reps	Weight	Reps	Weight

Muscle Group: Upper abdominals

Degree of Difficulty: Difficult

Lie on the floor and place your lower legs on top of a bench with your feet over the side. Position yourself close enough to the bench so your legs are at about a 45° angle. Put your hands behind your head and exhale as you pull your torso up as closely to your upper thighs as possible. Then you return to starting position and inhale. Do not swing your body up and down but concentrate on the abdominals and erectors to do the work.

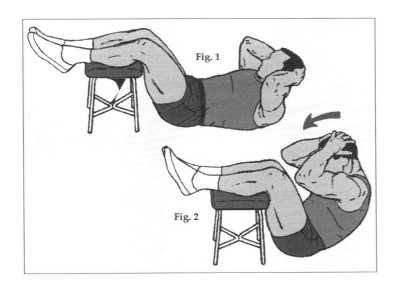

Sets/Reps: 3 sets of 10-30 reps

Date	Set One		Set Two		Set Three	
	Reps	Weight	Reps	Weight	Reps	Weight

Muscle Group: Lower abdominals

Degree of Difficulty: Intermediate

Lie on a flat bench with your legs off the end of the bench. Place your hands under your buttocks with your palms facing down. With your legs held straight in front of you, inhale and bend your knees while pulling your upper thighs into your midsection. Return to starting position and exhale. Concentrate on your lower abdominals during the exercise. Note that your lower legs are parallel to the floor at the halfway point of the exercise.

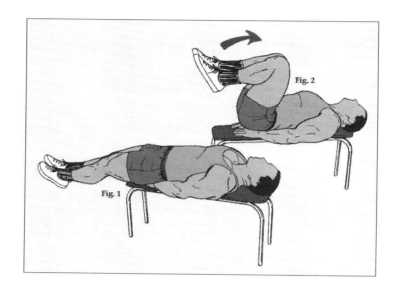

Sets/Reps: 3 sets of 10-30 reps

Date	Set One		Set Two		Set Three	
	Reps	Weight	Reps	Weight	Reps	Weight

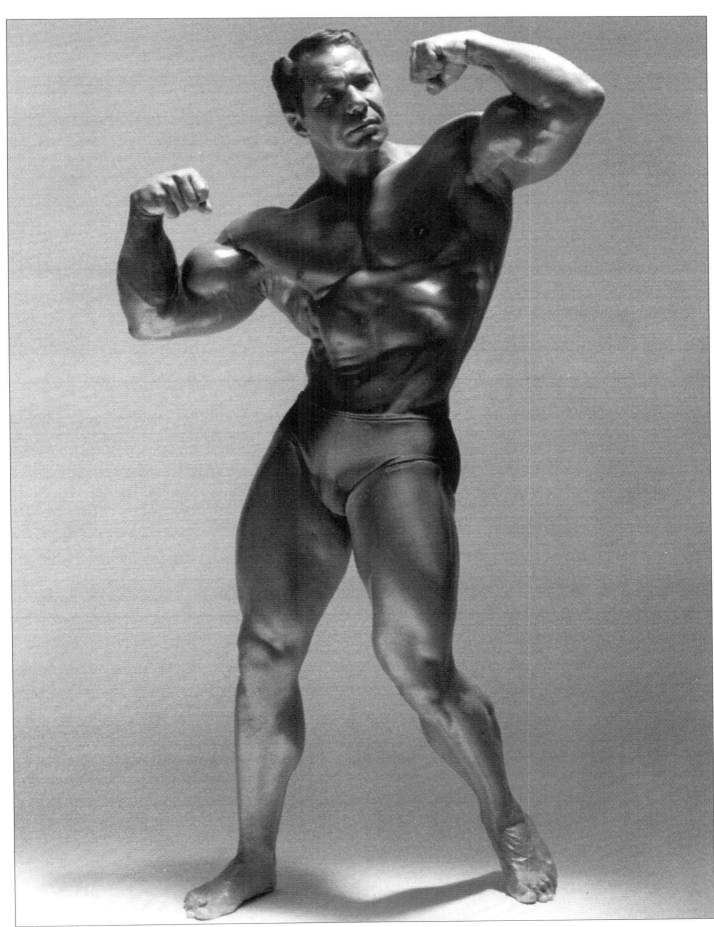

From any angle or pose Bill assumes, size, symmetry, proportions were all uniform. A gift from God and hard work.

Chapter 3

Month Two

Exercise	
1. Flat Footed Medium Stance Free Hand Squat	3 sets of 15-25 reps
2. Standing Toe Raise on Wall Calf Machine	3 sets of 20-25 reps
3. Bent Arm Lateral	3 sets of 10-12 reps
4. Medium Grip Straight Arm Barbell Pullover	3 sets of 10-12 reps
5. Seated Side Lateral Raise	3 sets of 10-12 reps
6. Wide Grip Front Lat Pull-Down	3 sets of 10-12 reps
7. Standing Close Grip Triceps Press Down on Lat Machine	3 sets of 10-12 reps
8. Standing Alternated Dumbbell Curl	3 sets of 10-12 reps
9. Dumbbell Side Bend	1 set of 25-50 reps
10. Bent Knee Sit-Up	1 set of 15-30 reps

In this second month of the beginner phase you will again train your entire body at each workout. The routine now consists of 10 exercises one more than last month. Since all the exercises have been changed, you will do an entirely new routine. Notice, however, that the order in which you train the respective body parts stays essentially the same as it was last month - legs, chest, deltoids, back, triceps, biceps and midsection. In months to come we'll alter the order for the sake of variety.

I want to emphasize some basic points to ensure that your training continues to be both productive and enjoyable. No workout program will make you a champion overnight, and no matter how much progress you make on a program, it does not mean much if you quit training because of boredom or burnout a few months down the road.

Keep in mind that you must make your training interesting, challenging and enjoyable; don't go over the line by pushing yourself to physical extremes, to the point where your workouts begin to seem more like mind destruction than bodybuilding.

If you are a beginner, remember, too, that you are still familiarizing yourself with the weights, the exercises and your body. Realize that you are building a foundation for what you hope will become a positive lifetime habit - a healthy, fitness lifestyle that will give you the body, strength and vitality you want. To lay that foundation properly, of course, you must first establish a positive relationship with the weight and your training. The best way to do that is to make your workouts fun. And if that's too much to ask, at least try to make the experience pleasant.

Don't get me wrong. It takes hard work and real dedication to build an outstanding physique, but there's a big difference between training hard and making the workouts so demanding the you exhaust your enthusiasm long before you come anywhere near perfecting your body. Most beginning bodybuilders - in fact, most people who train with weights have a tendency to overdo it rather than under do it, and the result is that far too many of them ultimately wind up saying, "To hell with it! What am I putting myself through this for?," and they quit training altogether. In my many years in bodybuilding and the gym business I've seen it happen more times than I care to remember. Don't let it happen to you.

One of the key points of my weight-training philosophy is that the training has to become a part of your daily regimen. You cannot back off from it. Your body loses strength at a rate of about 5 percent every 72 hours that you don't exercise, which is a very rapid regression. For example, if you work out for six months and then lay off for six months, all the gains and health benefits that you achieved will be gone.

To put it another way, in order for weight training to be something that continually pays you dividends, you have to continue putting something in the pot, so to speak, month after month, year after year. Your life has to revolve around some kind of fitness program in terms of training, eating habits, rest and so forth. You cannot rely on what you did six months or a year ago to keep you healthy and fit today. The dividends you earned from the training you did back then are all used up now. It's what you do today, what you plan to do tomorrow and what you do tomorrow that keep you healthy and fit not what you did six months or a year ago.

And that brings us back to the point that I always try

to hammer home: You must strive to make your training interesting, meaningful and enjoyable - actually make a conscious effort to do that - and you must make it something that you want to come back to day after day, month after month and year after year. I always try to leave the gym with a feeling that I have something in reserve so that I can return the next day and do it all again. I never try to "take out all the marbles" in one workout. I always leave with something in hand in terms of energy and strength so that I know that I can do a little bit better the next time I go to train. I suggest you do the same.

The Weight-Training Habit

You will notice that I haven't emphasized diet, weight loss or gain, aerobic exercise or other health factors like smoking or drinking in this program thus far. That's because I want you to get into the habit of weight training so that you can develop muscle tone, strength and the capacity to handle gradually increasing work loads. Our objective is not to revolutionize all of your habits overnight. In fact, if we tried, chances are it would be overkill and you might abandon your bodybuilding program almost before you got started. Therefore, we'll take one thing at a time, and the first objective is to get you into the habit of working out. With that as a foundation, or starting point, we can later go on to address the other aspects of a true fitness lifestyle.

Here are a few important tips for beginners:

- Rest when you feel the necessity. If you are feeling tired, cut back the work load or intensity of a given session. Decrease each exercise by one set or cut back on the weight or reps.
- Learn to focus on the body part you are training. When you are training a particular muscle, mentally concentrate on that muscle and make it do as much of the work as possible. Strict exercise form is a very important part of this.
- Take some photographs. This is a great way to monitor your progress as you continue training. Take some before shots in various poses from the front, side and back; both flexed and standing relaxed. Then periodically take additional photos and study the progress you have made. Remember, photos don't lie.
- Record your weight and take your measurements. This is another excellent way to evaluate your progress. Use a tailor's tape and measure your chest when it's expanded and normal, your waist, your

hips, your thighs, your calves and your upper arms. Take these same measurements again a few months later and compare.

Training Suggestions for Month 2

- Do this routine three times a week -- Monday, Wednesday and Friday, or Tuesday, Thursday and Saturday -- as you did last month. Use the off days for rest and recuperation.
- Since you progressed to three sets per exercise by the end of last month, I recommend that you continue with that number of sets -- except where the routine indicates otherwise. Since last month's workout didn't include any calf work, it's advisable that you start with only one set per workout on standing calf raises and build up to three sets. Your progression with that exercise might resemble the following:
  - Week 1: One set and minimum reps.
  - Week 2: Two sets and medium reps.
  - Week 3 and 4: Three sets and maximum reps.
- Use a poundage that's comfortable yet challenging for the indicated reps. At the beginning of this routine you'll have to do some experimentation to determine what weights you should use. Don't train to failure! The last rep should feel difficult but not impossible.
- As you continue training and your strength improves, the sets and reps will begin to feel easy with the poundages you've been using. Whenever you reach that point, increase the weight in the particular exercise until the last rep is difficult again. Always keep accurate records of your exercises, sets and reps from workout to workout, week to week and month to month. This will enable you to easily keep track of your progress from one poundage to the next rather than making the whole process haphazard. Don't get caught in the bind of always trying to top your last workout, however. Remember that the last rep should feel difficult, but it should not be an all-out effort.
- Concentrate on correct form on each exercise, mentally focus on the bodypart you're working.
- Rest for 30 seconds to two minutes between sets. If you feel any kind of unusual pain during your workout, check with a trainer. Of course, if you're just starting an exercise program, you should always check with a physician to ensure that you have no health problems that could make training dangerous.
- If three sets per exercise at the beginning of this

month seems a little too taxing or time consuming for you, feel free to go back to one or two sets and work up again. You may feel the need to ease off on the volume of work if you're a beginner, and this will allow you to regroup and work back up.

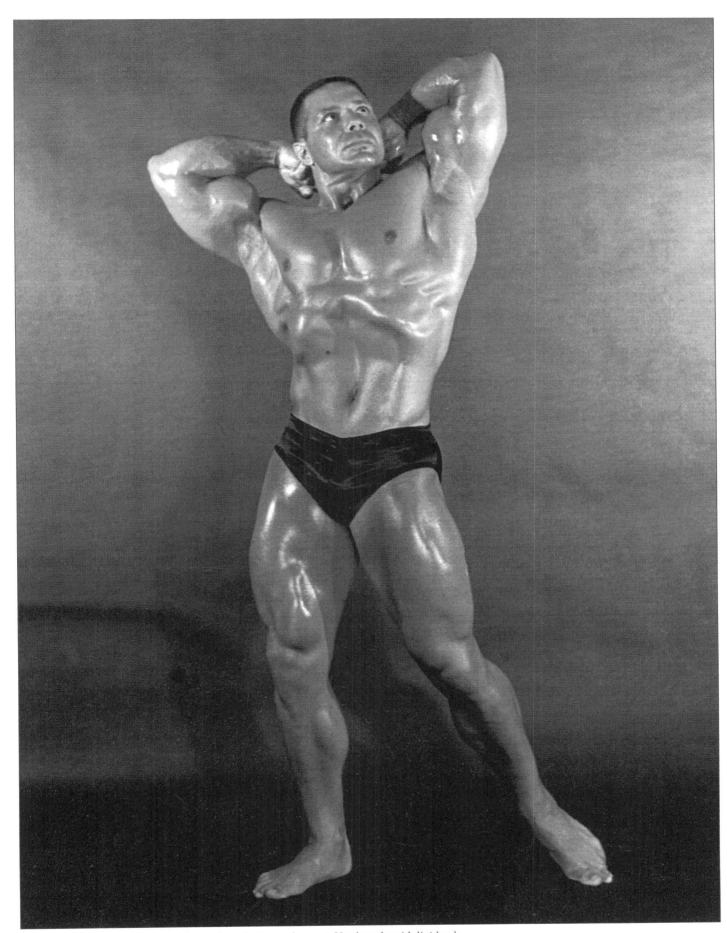

Pearl's chest was a weak point in his physique during early years. Hard work paid dividends.

Muscle Group: Upper thighs

Degree of Difficulty: Easy

Stand erect with your arms crossed over your chest. Keep your head up, back straight, and your feet planted firmly on the floor about sixteen inches apart. Inhale and squat down until your upper thighs are parallel with the floor and exhale. Your head should remain up, back straight, and your knees slightly out to the sides. Return to starting position and exhale.

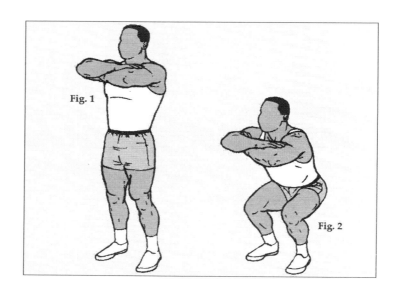

Sets/Reps: 3 sets of 15-25 reps

Date	Set One		Set Two		Set Three	
	Reps	Weight	Reps	Weight	Reps	Weight

Muscle Group: Main calf muscles
Degree of Difficulty: Intermediate

Position your shoulders under the extended portion of a wall calf machine. Stand erect and place the balls of your feet on the footpad that is directly below the extended portion of the machine. Keep your back straight, head up and legs locked during the entire exercise. Do not let your hips move backward and forward while performing the exercise. Lower your heels to the lowest possible comfortable position. Inhale and raise up on your toes as high as possible. Hold this position for a short period and return to starting position and exhale. If you turn your toes out and heels in, it will affect the inner calf more. If you keep your feet straight, it will affect the main calf muscle more. If you turn your toes in and heels out, it will affect the outside of the calf more.

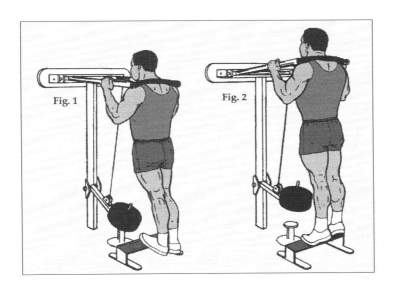

Fig. 1   Fig. 2

Sets/Reps: 3 sets of 20-25 reps

Date	Set One		Set Two		Set Three	
	Reps	Weight	Reps	Weight	Reps	Weight

Muscle Group: Outer pectorals

Degree of Difficulty: Intermediate

Lie on a flat bench with the dumbbells together at arm's length above the shoulders The palms of the hands should be facing each other. Slowly lower the dumbbells to the down position so the dumbbells are approximately even with the chest but out about ten inches from each side of the chest. Notice that the elbows are drawn downwards and back so they are in line with the ears. The forearms are slightly out of a vertical position. The press back to starting position is done by using the same arc as in letting the dumbbells down. Inhale at the beginning of the exercise and exhale at the finish.

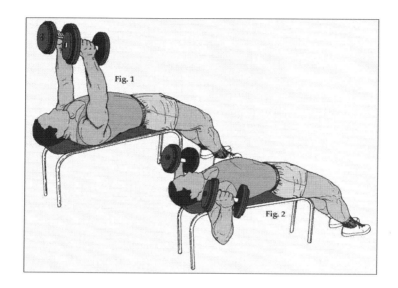

Sets/Reps: 3 sets of 10-12 reps

Date	Set One		Set Two		Set Three	
	Reps	Weight	Reps	Weight	Reps	Weight

Muscle Group: Pectorals and rib cage
Degree of Difficulty: Intermediate

Lie supine on a flat bench with your head at the end of the bench. With a barbell held at arm's length above the chest and a hand spacing about twenty-four inches apart, take a deep breath and lower the barbell in a semicircle past the chest and head until it is lowered to a position behind your head that brings no discomfort to the shoulder area. It is possible you may go nearly to the floor if the bench is not too high. From the low position, return the barbell to starting position still keeping the elbows in a locked position. Exhale as you reach the starting position. Keep the head down, your chest high, breathe deeply and do not raise your hips off the bench.

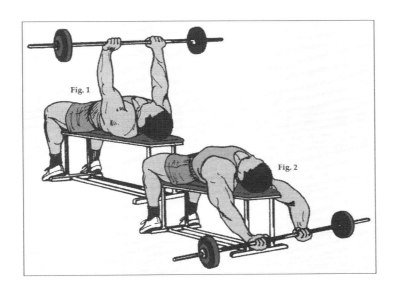

Sets/Reps: 3 sets of 10-12 reps

Date	Set One		Set Two		Set Three	
	Reps	Weight	Reps	Weight	Reps	Weight

Muscle Group: Front and outer deltoids

Degree of Difficulty: Intermediate

Sit on the edge of a bench with your legs fairly close together and dumbbells at arm's length, palms facing in toward the thighs. Slowly raise the dumbbells to a position a little above shoulder height, pause, then lower them back to starting position. Keep the arms straight throughout the execution of the exercise. Inhale when raising the dumbbells and exhale as they are lowered.

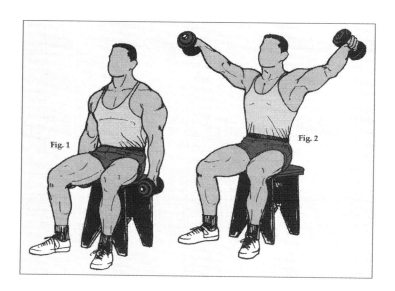

Fig. 1　　Fig. 2

Sets/Reps: 3 sets of 10-12 reps

	Set One		Set Two		Set Three	
Date	Reps	Weight	Reps	Weight	Reps	Weight

WIDE GRIP FRONT LAT PULL-DOWN

Muscle Group: Upper lats

Degree of Difficulty: Intermediate

Place your hands on a lat machine about thirty-six inches apart. Kneel down on your knees until you are supporting the weight stack with your arms while they are extended overhead. Inhale and pull the bar straight down until it is even with your upper chest. Return to starting position and exhale.

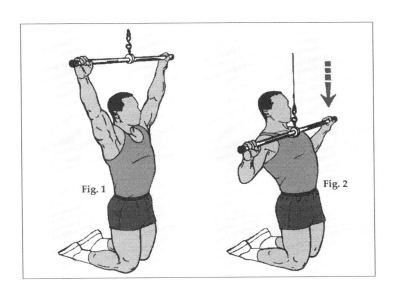

Sets/Reps: 3 sets of 10-12 reps

Date	Set One		Set Two		Set Three	
	Reps	Weight	Reps	Weight	Reps	Weight

Muscle Group: Outer triceps

Degree of Difficulty: Intermediate

Stand erect in front of a lat machine with your feet about sixteen inches apart and your back straight. Grasp the lat machine bar with both hands using a palms down grip about eight inches apart. Bring your upper arms to your sides and keep them there throughout the exercise. Your forearms and biceps should be touching as you inhale and then press the bar down in a semicircular motion to arm's length. Return to starting position using a similar path, in a controlled manner, and exhale. Be sure to keep tension on your triceps while pressing down and returning to starting position.

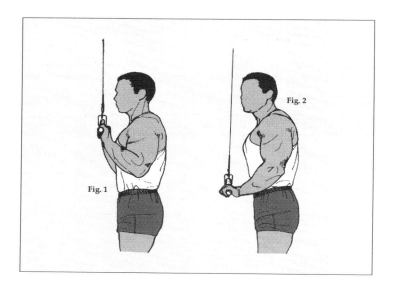

Sets/Reps: 3 sets of 10-12 reps

Date	Set One		Set Two		Set Three	
	Reps	Weight	Reps	Weight	Reps	Weight

Muscle Group: Biceps

Degree of Difficulty: Intermediate

Grasp a dumbbell in each hand and stand erect with your back straight, head up and feet about sixteen inches apart. With the dumbbells hanging at arm's length from your sides, palms facing in, inhale and curl the dumbbell in your right hand up past your right thigh and then turn your palm up and keep it in this up position throughout the exercise until you are lowering the weight and again near your upper thigh before turning the palm in again and exhaling. Do a repetition with your right arm and then one with your left arm. Continue going from right to left until the prescribed number of repetitions are completed.

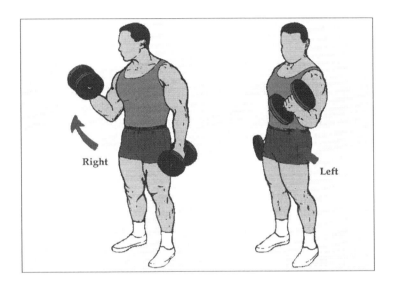

Sets/Reps: 3 sets of 10-12 reps

	Set One		Set Two		Set Three	
Date	Reps	Weight	Reps	Weight	Reps	Weight

Muscle Group: Obliques

Degree of Difficulty: Intermediate

Stand erect with your feet about sixteen inches apart and grasp a dumbbell in your right hand. Your palm will be facing your upper thigh. Place your left hand on your left oblique. Inhale and bend to the right as far as possible and then bend to the left as far as possible and exhale. You will perform the prescribed number of repetitions and then change the weight to the left hand and repeat the movement. You must remember to keep your back straight and your head up or you will bend too far forward.

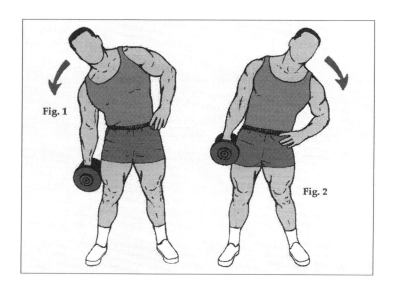

Fig. 1

Fig. 2

Sets/Reps: 1 set of 25-50 reps

Date	Set One					
	Reps	Weight				

BENT KNEE SIT-UP

Muscle Group: Upper abdominals
Degree of Difficulty: Intermediate

Sit down on a sit-up board and hook your feet under the strap. With your knees bent to about a 45° angle, put your hands behind your head and place your chin on your chest. This will keep a slight bow to your back. From this position, inhale and lie back until your lower back touches the board. Exhale as you return to starting position.

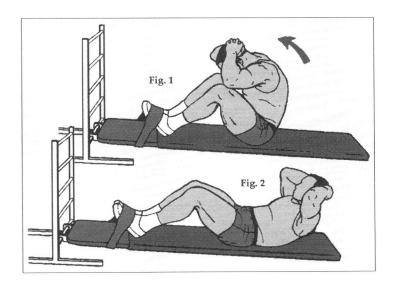

Sets/Reps: 1 set of 15-30 reps

	Set One				
Date	Reps	Weight			

Chapter 4

Month 3

Exercise	
1. Incline Lateral	3-4 sets of 10-12 reps
2. Hand on Bench One Arm Dumbbell Rowing	3-4 sets of 10-12 reps
3. Standing Military Press	3-4 sets of 10-12 reps
4. Lying Supine Close Grip Barbell Triceps Curl to Chin	3-4 sets of 10-12 reps
5. Seated Dumbbell Curl	3-4 sets of 10-12 reps
6. Heels Elevated Wide Stance Barbell Hack Squat	3-4 sets of 10-12 reps
7. Free Hand Front Lunge	3-4 sets of 10-12 reps
8. Seated Toe Raise on Seated Calf Machine	3-4 sets of 20-25 reps
9. Bend to the Opposite Foot	1 set of 20-30 reps
10. Bent Knee Sit Up	1 set of 15-30 reps

This month we change the order in which you train the various muscle groups. For the past two months, you will recall, you worked legs first, followed by chest, deltoids, back, arms and midsection.

In addition, of course, you perform an almost entirely new routine - only one exercise, the bent-knee sit-up, is carried over from last month - and in the last two weeks you increase the number of sets per exercise to four from the previous high of three.

Another thing that's different about this month's workout is that it does not include a movement that's classified as a direct deltoid exercise, such as the seated side laterals that you did last month. Even so, your delts get significant although indirect stress in the first exercise of this routine, incline laterals. Remember that it's impossible to work your chest without working your delts.

More important is the fact that the military press, which is the third exercise in this routine, is one of the most difficult shoulder, or deltoid, exercises you can do. Because it works both the traps and shoulders, it is not regarded as strictly a deltoid exercise. Under the circumstances, however, I'd be reluctant to recommend any more delt work than you are going to be getting here.

Indeed, the military press is so demanding that you may find yourself arching your back from the effort on the last few reps. This can aggravate any low-back instability you may have. If you have a history of low-back problems, and many people do, you can do this exercise seated. That will take the pressure off your back - and actually make the movement seem harder, since you cannot cheat by arching your back and getting your lag and hip muscles into the action as you press the barbell up. You may also want to

wear a lifting belt to give your back added support.

And now that you have presumably been training consistently for two months and have established something of a foundation with your weight training - even if you are a beginner - let me address a point that's crucial to your bodybuilding progress. As you know, I have emphasized over and over again in this program that you should not train to failure. Don't get me wrong - in no way, shape or form am I suggesting that you coast through your workouts. The last rep of each set should not be an all-out effort, but it should be a challenge.

Another very important point is that you should try to do a little more work every time you go into the gym. Don't try for a lot more, but make some type of increase in intensity or work load each time so you are not just maintaining. Remember that this is a progressive-resistance weight-training program. Only by increasing your intensity or work load from week to week and month to month will you see results. Besides, as you continue training and increase your strength, it's only common sense that you try to do more. Otherwise, a workout that seemed challenging a few weeks ago will now seem less so, and your progress will, consequently, slow down.

The stronger a muscle becomes, the more work you must give it in order for it to keep increasing in size, strength and tone. That's the very essence and the underlying principle of progressive-resistance training. Indeed, it's the principle of any type of physical training - you push the body, give it an opportunity to rest, recuperate and consolidate its fitness gains and then push it again. Runners do it, cyclists do it, and bodybuilders do it. Simply put, it's the way all athletes go from a lower level to a higher level of conditioning, whatever the sport.

Naturally, there will be days when you go into the gym and you may feel tired or under the weather for some reason. On those days you may decide - and wisely so - to cut back on the intensity or work load. Generally speaking, however, try to keep increasing the effort you subject your muscles to from workout to workout. It will pay off in the weeks and months to come. I guarantee it.

A Simple Answer to a Common Problem

Bodybuilders sometimes say to me, "Bill, when I am doing several sets of an exercise, I often have trouble completing the full number of reps in the final sets with the weight I started out with. If I can somehow complete all the reps on the last few sets with that weight, it's a struggle and my exercise form goes all to pieces. What should I do?"

The answer is simple, though it goes against the grain of what most bodybuilders have a tendency to do under the circumstances: You should cut back the poundages on the last few sets of an exercise in order to complete the prescribed number of reps - actually decrease the weight you are using so you can continue to use correct exercise form and stay within the don't-train-to-failure guideline.

Of course, if you are like most bodybuilders, your ego gets in the way as you struggle to complete all the reps in the last set or two, and the idea that's running through your brain is, "I'll be damned if I am going to decrease the weight I am using!".

That's the natural tendency, but it's important to clearly and objectively keep in mind the bigger picture, which is your overall training philosophy and what you are trying to accomplish.

I always say, You control the weights; they don't control you. If you don't give yourself the freedom to adjust your poundages upward or downward to complete your workout in the manner in which you set out to do it, the result is that the weights win and you lose. Decrease the weight if necessary on the last few sets of an exercise so that you not only complete the required number of reps, but you also do it with correct form.

Training Suggestions for Month 3

- For best results do this routine three times a week - Monday, Wednesday and Friday or Tuesday, Thursday and Saturday. Use the off days for rest and recuperation.
- Last month you progressed to three sets per exercise for most of the movements. This month I suggest that on exercises 1 through 8 you do three sets and the minimum reps, 10, for the first two weeks and four sets and the maximum reps, 12, for the last two.

- On the two midsection exercises that conclude this routine, do only one set per workout and increase the reps from workout to workout. Start out at the low end of the rep range at the beginning of the month and gradually build up until you're at the high end of the rep range at the end of the month. Since you already worked through this rep buildup last month with the bent-knee sit-up, I recommend that you repeat the sequence but with the bench at a slightly steeper angle so the intensity is greater.

- Do not train to failure. The last rep should feel difficult but should not be an all-out effort. At the beginning of this routine you'll have to experiment to determine what poundages you should use in order to make the last rep or two challenging but not impossible.

- Increase the poundage on each exercise as warranted by your strength increases. Remember, you want to make the last rep of each set challenging. Make sure you keep accurate records of your exercises, sets and reps from workout to workout, week to week and month to month. This will enable you to easily keep track of your progress from one poundage to the next rather than making the whole process haphazard.

- Concentrate on correct form when doing each exercise, and mentally focus on the bodypart you're working.

- Rest for 30 seconds to two minutes between sets. If you feel any kind of unusual pain during your workout, consult with a trainer. Of course, if you're just starting a training program, you should always check with a physician to ensure that you have no health problems that could make training dangerous.

- If three sets per exercise at the beginning of this month seems too much for you or is too time consuming, feel free to go back to fewer sets and work up again. Likewise, if you're not felling up to par during a given workout, don't hesitate to cut back on your sets. Sometimes it's necessary to ease off the volume of work, regroup and work back up - and the intelligent bodybuilder knows when and where to do this. Generally speaking, however, the idea is to increase the intensity and volume of your work load gradually. That's what you're aiming for and what will give you the best results.

Muscle Group: Upper pectorals

Degree of Difficulty: Intermediate

Use a hand position on the dumbbells similar to that of holding a barbell. Start with the dumbbells together at arm's length above the shoulders. Slowly lower them to the down position so the dumbbells are approximately even with the chest but about ten inches from each side of the chest. Notice that the elbows are drawn downwards and back so they are in line with the ears. The forearms are slightly out of a vertical position. The press back to starting position is done by using the same arc as in letting the dumbbells down. Inhale at the beginning of the exercise and exhale at the finish.

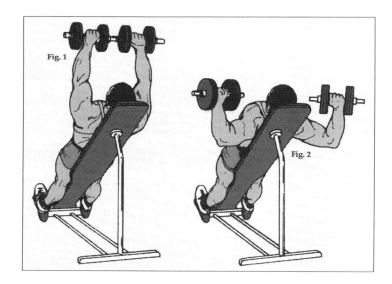

Sets/Reps: 3-4 sets of 10-12 reps

Date	Set One		Set Two		Set Three		Set Four	
	Reps	Weight	Reps	Weight	Reps	Weight	Reps	Weight

HAND ON BENCH ONE ARM DUMBBELL ROWING

Muscle Group: Upper and lower lats
Degree of Difficulty: Intermediate

Place a dumbbell on the floor in front of a bench. Put your left leg back, keeping your left knee locked. Bend the right leg slightly as you bend down and grasp the dumbbell with your left hand, using a palms in grip. Place your right hand on the bench and lock the elbow. With the dumbbell in your left hand hanging straight down and off the floor about six inches, inhale and pull the dumbbell straight up to the side of your chest, keeping your arm in close. Return to starting position and exhale. Do the prescribed number of repetitions on the right side and then change positions to the left side doing the same number of repetitions. Be sure the dumbbell does not touch the floor once the exercise has begun.

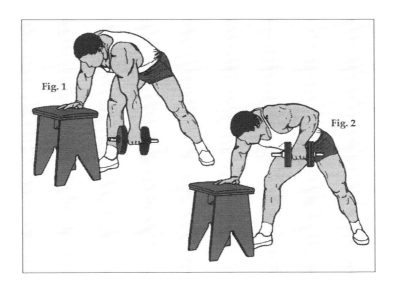

Sets/Reps: 3-4 sets of 10-12 reps

Date	Set One		Set Two		Set Three		Set Four	
	Reps	Weight	Reps	Weight	Reps	Weight	Reps	Weight

STANDING MILITARY PRESS

Muscle Group: Front and outer deltoids
Degree of Difficulty: Intermediate

This is the standard military press. Clean the weight to the chest. Lock the legs and hips solidly. This will give you a solid platform from which to push. Keep the elbows in slightly and under the bar, press the weight overhead, lock the arms out. When lowering the barbell to the upper chest, be sure it rests on the chest and is not held with the arms. If the chest is held high, it will give you a nice shelf on which to place the barbell and to push from. Inhale before the press and exhale when lowering the barbell.

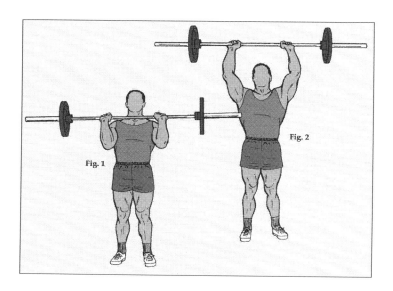

Sets/Reps: 3-4 sets of 10-12 reps

Date	Set One		Set Two		Set Three		Set Four	
	Reps	Weight	Reps	Weight	Reps	Weight	Reps	Weight

Muscle Group: Triceps
Degree of Difficulty: Intermediate

Hold a barbell with both hands using a palms down grip about six inches apart. Lie on a flat bench with your head over the end of the bench pointing downward towards the floor. Press the barbell to arm's length keeping it in line with your shoulders. Inhale and lower the barbell straight down in a semicircular motion by bending your arms at the elbows but keeping your upper arms vertical throughout the exercise. The barbell should be lowered to your chin and your forearms and biceps should touch. Press the barbell back to starting position using the same path and exhale.

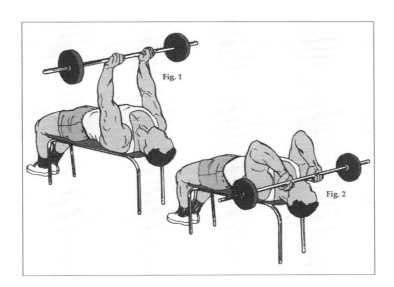

Sets/Reps: 3-4 sets of 10-12 reps

	Set One		Set Two		Set Three		Set Four	
Date	Reps	Weight	Reps	Weight	Reps	Weight	Reps	Weight

SEATED DUMBBELL CURL

Muscle Group: Biceps

Degree of Difficulty: Intermediate

Hold a dumbbell in each hand and sit at the end of a flat bench with your back straight, head up and feet planted firmly on the floor. With the dumbbells hanging at arm's length at your sides, with your palms in, inhale and curl the dumbbells up to the height of your shoulders. As you commence the curl and the dumbbells are past your thighs, then turn your palms-up and keep them in this position throughout the exercise until you are lowering the weights and again near your upper thighs before turning your palms in again and exhaling. Keep your upper arms in close to your sides and concentrate on your biceps raising and lowering the weights.

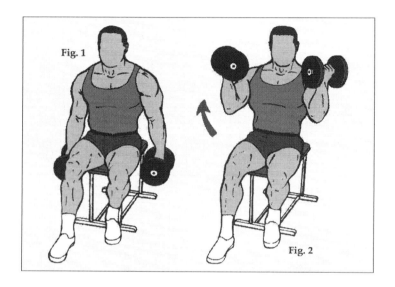

Sets/Reps: 3-4 sets of 10-12 reps

Date	Set One		Set Two		Set Three		Set Four	
	Reps	Weight	Reps	Weight	Reps	Weight	Reps	Weight

Muscle Group: Inner thighs
Degree of Difficulty: Intermediate

Place a barbell at arm's length behind you keeping the bar tucked in solidly against your body where your buttocks and upper thighs meet. Use a palms up facing to the rear grip with your hand spacing about the width of your hips. Now, turn your wrist up to lock the bar into an even more solid position. The bar is to remain solidly against your upper thighs and lower buttocks during the entire exercise. It is not to slide up and down on your leg biceps. Keep your head up and your eyes staring upward at about a 45° angle. Keep your back straight and your feet on a 2x4 piece of wood about thirty inches apart. Inhale and squat down until your upper thighs are parallel with the floor. Your head should remain up, eyes looking upward, back straight and knees pointing outward. Return to starting position and exhale.

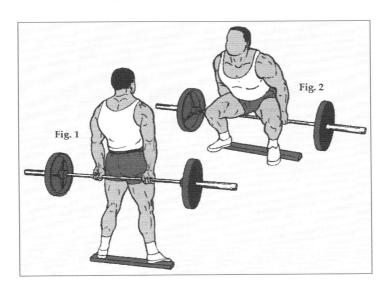

Sets/Reps: 3-4 sets of 10-12 reps

Date	Set One		Set Two		Set Three		Set Four	
	Reps	Weight	Reps	Weight	Reps	Weight	Reps	Weight

FREE HAND FRONT LUNGE

Muscle Group: Thighs and thigh biceps

Degree of Difficulty: Intermediate

Stand erect with your hands placed on your hips. Keep your head up, back straight and feet planted firmly on the floor about fourteen inches apart. Inhale and step forward as far as possible with your right leg until your upper right thigh is almost parallel with the floor. Your left leg should be held as straight as possible not bending the knee any more than is necessary. From this position, step back to starting position and exhale. Do the prescribed number of repetitions with your right leg and then repeat the same number of repetitions with your left leg.

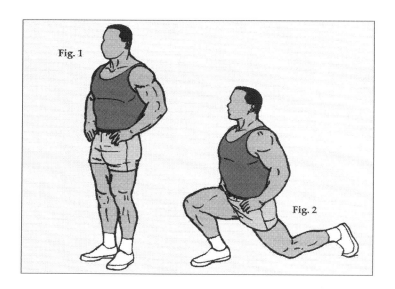

Sets/Reps: 3-4 sets of 10-12 reps

Date	Set One		Set Two		Set Three		Set Four	
	Reps	Weight	Reps	Weight	Reps	Weight	Reps	Weight

SEATED TOE RAISE ON SEATED CALF MACHINE

Muscle Group: Main calf muscles

Degree of Difficulty: Intermediate

Sit on the seat of a seated calf machine and place your upper thighs, just above your knees, under the leg pad. Place the bails of your feet on the footpad that is directly below the leg pad. Raise up on your toes and release the safety stops. Lower your heels to the lowest possible comfortable position. Inhale and raise up on your toes as high as possible. Hold this position for a short period and return to starting position and exhale. If you turn your toes out and heels in, it will affect the inner calf more. If you keep your feet straight, it will affect the main calf muscle more. If you turn your toes in and heels out, it will affect the outside of the calf more.

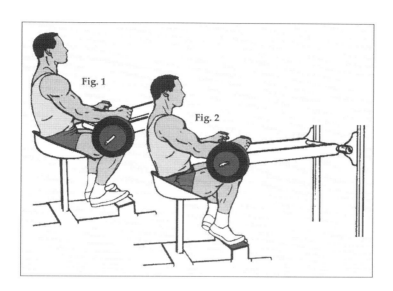

Sets/Reps: 3-4 sets of 20-25 reps

Date	Set One		Set Two		Set Three		Set Four	
	Reps	Weight	Reps	Weight	Reps	Weight	Reps	Weight

BEND TO OPPOSITE FOOT

Muscle Group: Rear obliques

Degree of Difficulty: Intermediate

Stand erect with your feet about sixteen inches apart. Grasp a dumbbell in your right hand with your palms facing in. Place your left hand on your upper left thigh. Place your right arm across your waist so the dumbbell will be in line with your left thigh. Exhale and bend downward until the dumbbell nearly touches your left foot. Return to starting position and exhale. Perform the prescribed number of repetitions before changing the dumbbell over to the left hand to repeat the right movement.

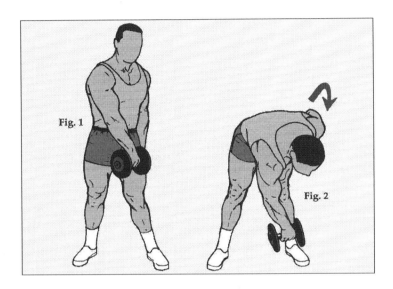

Sets/Reps: 1 set of 20-30 reps

Date	Set One					
	Reps	Weight				

BENT KNEE SIT-UP

Muscle Group: Upper abdominals

Degree of Difficulty: Intermediate

Sit down on a sit-up board and hook your feet under the strap. With your knees bent to about a 45° angle, put your hands behind your head and place your chin on your chest. This will keep a slight bow to your back. From this position, inhale and lie back until your lower back touches the board. Exhale as you return to starting position.

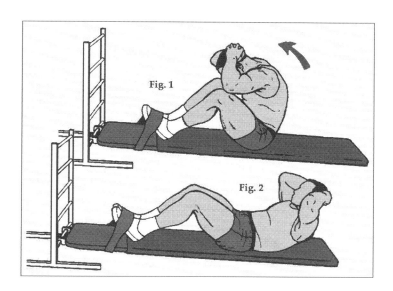

Sets/Reps: 1 set of 15-30 reps

Date	Set One					
	Reps	Weight				

Chapter 5

Month 4

Exercise	
1. Decline Dumbbell Fly	3-4 sets of 10-12 reps
2. Seated Two Arm Low Lat Pull-In	3-4 sets of 10-12 reps
3. Bent Over Low Pulley Rear Deltoid Raise	3-4 sets of 10-12 reps
4. Standing Bent Over One Dumbbell Triceps Extension	3-4 sets of 10-12 reps
5. Incline Dumbbell Curl	3-4 sets of 10-12 reps
6. Flat Footed Close Stance Barbell Hack Squat	3-4 sets of 10-12 reps
7. Thigh Biceps Curl on Leg Extension Machine	3-4 sets of 10-12 reps
8. Seated Lower Pad Toe Raise on Universal Type Leg Press Machine	3-4 sets of 20-25 reps
9. Bent Knee Sit Up	1 set of 15-30 reps
10. Incline Leg Pull-In	1 set of 15-30 reps

One of the keys to success in bodybuilding -- and in life itself, for that matter -- is to have clear and definite goals. The trick is to set a series of short-term goals that lead to a long-term goal. If you haven't already done so, start setting some short-term bodybuilding goals that you know you can achieve, and once you have reached them, set new goals that will be slightly more challenging and will bring you that much closer to your long-term target.

And what is your long-term goal? Get clear on that point, and use your long-term goal as both an orienting vision and an aspiration in your day-to-day training. Progress is made through goal setting. If you don't have goals, your training lacks purpose and meaning. To put it another way, how can you expect to get to your destination if you don't know where you are going?

There are literally hundreds of training goals that you can set. As you continue with this program, one of your goals might simply be to conscientiously perform each month's routine, constantly striving to do a little better at each workout, pushing yourself a little more each time yet being careful not to overdo it. Bodyweight could be a goal - you may want to set goals pertaining to how much muscle mass you want to gain or body fat you want to lose. You could target the arm, waist, thigh and/or calf measurements you hope to achieve in a certain period of time or the overall appearance you want to project. At the end of six months, for instance, you may want to have a trim, well-defined waistline.

Other possible achievements to aim for include how many pants sizes -- or dress sizes -- you want to drop, how much stronger and more energetic you want to become, how much you want to tighten up your diet as you tone and tighten your body and how much aerobic exercise you want to do as you continue your weight-training program and the tone and shape of your body improve. There are also any number of health goals you can target; for example, to stop smoking, avoid excessive drinking or decrease your cholesterol count.

It's up to you to decide what you want to achieve. The important thing is to set goals you can reach and put time limits on them. Then promise yourself that you will reach those goals -- and keep your commitment. Every time you reach a goal, you chalk up another success experience and put yourself in a position, physically and psychologically, to strive for something even more challenging. With one success building on another, pretty soon you will surprise even yourself by how far you have progressed and what you have achieved.

Remember that the key is to set short -- term goals that are reasonable and attainable. There's nothing wrong with having a big dream in life and having challenging goals to take you there, but the key to success in anything is to rehearse success rather than rehearse failure. So make your goals difficult but achievable, and your training will be a series of positive experiences leading to more positive experiences, which ultimately translates to success in anybody's book.

Basic vs. Refinement Exercises

Generally speaking, when you are a beginning bodybuilder, you are trying to lay a foundation for what will become an outstanding physique, and when you are an advanced bodybuilder, you are trying to refine and polish that physique.

I am sometimes asked, "Are there certain exercises that only advanced bodybuilders should do?".

My answer is no. I think that anytime you are working a muscle through a complete contraction to extension from all possible angles and the exercise does not cause unnatural pain, it is beneficial for the body - whatever your training experience or stature as a bodybuilder. There is no such thing as an exercise that is for advanced bodybuilders only or, conversely, for beginning bodybuilders only. That is silly. As long as you can do it through a full range of motion and it does not cause unnatural pain, it is beneficial.

Which brings me to a second question I am sometimes asked - "Shouldn't beginning bodybuilders focus on certain basic exercises and then wait until they reach an advanced level to incorporate a greater selection of exercises to refine the physique?".

This is probably quite true, but let's not forget that it is the basics that have gotten advanced bodybuilders to where they are today. When we talk about basic exercises, we are talking about exercises that bring the most muscle and mass into play; for example, squats. This is an excellent exercise because it brings more muscle fibers into play than almost any other exercise you can do. There are other basic movements, such as military presses, bench presses and barbell curls, that are good foundation exercises to build on because they bring a lot of muscle fibers into play.

Yes, as you become a more advanced bodybuilder, you can and should do a greater range of exercises to refine you physique, but this does not mean that you should not do the basic movements as well. It is interesting to note that I included the medium-grip bench press in the first month of the beginner phase, and you will be doing this very same exercise again in the next to the last month during the advanced phase. Now you know why.

Training Suggestions for Month 4

- For best results do this routine three times a week - Monday, Wednesday and Friday or Tuesday, Thursday and Saturday. Use the off days for rest and recuperation.
- Last month you progressed to four sets per exercise for most of the movements. This month I suggest that you go back to three sets for the first week, then do four sets per exercise during the last three weeks.
- On the two midsection exercises that conclude this routine, do only one set per workout, gradually increasing the reps so you reach the upper end of the range by month's end.

- Do not train to failure! The last rep should feel difficult but should not be an all-out effort. At the beginning of this routine you'll have to experiment to determine the poundages that will fit the bill.
- Increase the poundages as you get stronger. Remember, you want to make the last rap of each set challenging. Keep accurate records of your sets and reps from workout to workout so you can easily keep track of your progress from one poundage to the next rather than relying on memory.
- Concentrate on correct form when doing each exercise, and mentally focus on the bodypart you're working.
- Rest for 30 seconds to two minutes between sets. If you feel any kind of unusual pain during your workout, consult with a trainer. Of course, if you're just starting a training program, you should always check with a physician to ensure that you have no health problems that could make training dangerous.

DECLINE DUMBBELL FLY

Muscle Group: Lower pectorals
Degree of Difficulty: Intermediate

Lie on a decline bench with two light dumbbells at arm's length above the shoulders with the palms of the hands facing each other. Keeping the arms as straight as possible, lower the dumbbells out to each side of the chest but slightly back so they are nearly in line with your ears. From this position return the weights back above the chest using the same path in which you used originally. Exhale as you reach the top position. You must breathe deeply, hold your chest high, keep your head on the bench and concentrate on the pectorals.

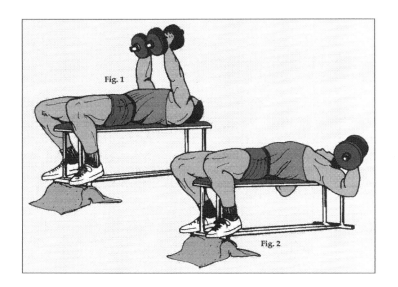

Sets/Reps: 3-4 sets of 10-12 reps

	Set One		Set Two		Set Three		Set Four	
Date	Reps	Weight	Reps	Weight	Reps	Weight	Reps	Weight

Muscle Group: Lower lats

Degree of Difficulty: Intermediate

Sit on the floor in front of a low pulley and place your feet against an object that will enable you to support the weight stacks with both arms as you grasp the pulley handles while seated in a bent-forward position. You must maintain this bent-forward position throughout the entire exercise. Do not bend backwards and forwards at the waist. Inhale and pull the cables directly to the sides of your chest just below the pectorals. Let the weight stacks back to starting position and exhale.

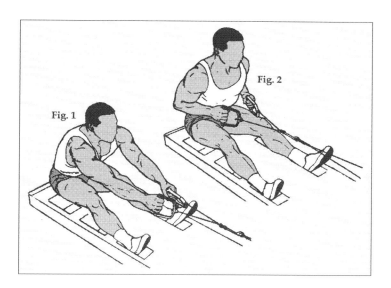

Sets/Reps: 3-4 sets of 10-12 reps

	Set One		Set Two		Set Three		Set Four	
Date	Reps	Weight	Reps	Weight	Reps	Weight	Reps	Weight

Muscle Group: Rear deltoids

Degree of Difficulty: Difficult

Face a wall pulley with the left side of your body and grasp the low handle of the wall pulley with your right hand. Step out away from the pulley so that you are supporting the weight stack with your right arm. Bend at the waist until your upper body is nearly parallel to the floor. Use your left arm to help support your upper body by placing it on your left thigh just above the knee. Keep your right elbow locked and your arm as straight as possible as you pull the weight up and out in a semicircular motion until your right arm is even in height to the right shoulder. Concentrate on having your right hand in line with your right ear at the top of the exercise. Inhale as you raise the weight and exhale as you lower the weight. You must do both the right side and the left side to constitute a set.

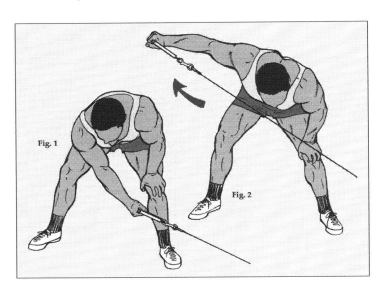

Sets/Reps: 3-4 sets of 10-12 reps

Date	Set One		Set Two		Set Three		Set Four	
	Reps	Weight	Reps	Weight	Reps	Weight	Reps	Weight

STANDING BENT OVER ONE DUMBBELL TRICEPS EXTENSION

Muscle Group: Triceps

Degree of Difficulty: Intermediate

Hold a dumbbell in your right hand with your palms facing in. Bend at the waist until your upper body is parallel with the floor. Draw your right upper arm to your side and keep your lower arm vertical. Inhale and press the dumbbell back in a semicircular motion until your entire arm is parallel with the floor. Hold the dumbbell at the top position for a short period to contract the triceps muscle and then slowly lower the weight back to starting position and exhale. Do the prescribed number of repetitions on the right side and then change positions doing the same number of repetitions on the left side.

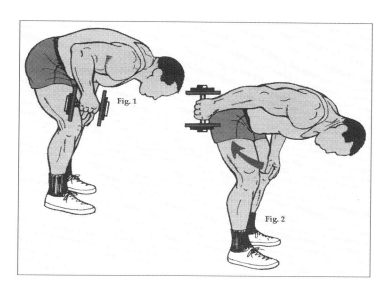

Sets/Reps: 3-4 sets of 10-12 reps

Date	Set One		Set Two		Set Three		Set Four	
	Reps	Weight	Reps	Weight	Reps	Weight	Reps	Weight

INCLINE DUMBBELL CURL

Muscle Group: Biceps

Degree of Difficulty: Intermediate

Hold a dumbbell in each hand and lie back on an incline bench with your head up and feet on the footpads. With the dumbbells hanging at arm's length at your sides, with your palms in, inhale and curl the dumbbells up to the height of your shoulders. As you commence the curl and the dumbbells are past your thighs, then turn your palms-up and keep them in this position throughout the exercise until you are lowering the weights and again near your upper thighs before turning your palms in again and exhaling. Keep your upper arms in close to your sides and concentrate or your biceps raising and lowering the weights.

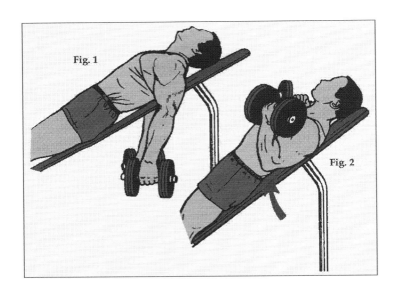

Sets/Reps: 3-4 sets of 10-12 reps

Date	Set One		Set Two		Set Three		Set Four	
	Reps	Weight	Reps	Weight	Reps	Weight	Reps	Weight

Muscle Group: Outer thighs

Degree of Difficulty: Difficult

Place a barbell at arm's length behind you keeping the bar tucked in solidly against your body where your buttocks and upper thighs meet. Use a palms facing to the rear grip with your hand spacing about the width of your hips. Now, turn your wrist up to lock the bar into an even more solid position. The bar is to remain solidly against your upper thighs and lower buttocks during the entire exercise. It is not to slide up and down on your leg biceps. Keep your head up and your eyes staring upward at about a 45° angle. Keep your back straight and feet planted firmly on the floor about eight inches apart. Inhale and squat down until your upper thighs are parallel with the floor. Your head should remain up, eyes looking upward, back straight and knees close together. Return to starting position and exhale.

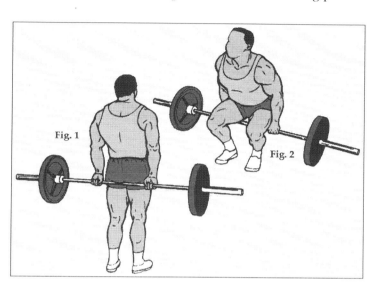

Fig. 1   Fig. 2

Sets/Reps: 3-4 sets of 10-12 reps

Date	Set One		Set Two		Set Three		Set Four	
	Reps	Weight	Reps	Weight	Reps	Weight	Reps	Weight

THIGH BICEPS CURL ON LEG EXTENSION MACHINE

Muscle Group: Thigh biceps

Degree of Difficulty: Intermediate

Lie face down on a leg extension machine with your feet to the front. Straighten your legs and place your heels under the top foot pads. Hold on to the front of the machine for support. Inhale and curl your legs up until your lower and upper legs come together. Return to starting position and exhale.

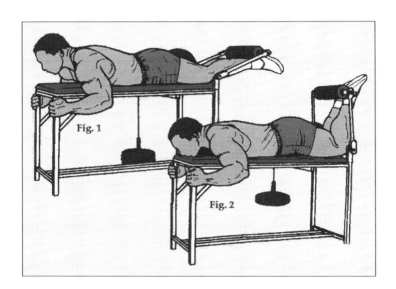

Sets/Reps: 3-4 sets of 10-12 reps

Date	Set One		Set Two		Set Three		Set Four	
	Reps	Weight	Reps	Weight	Reps	Weight	Reps	Weight

SEATED LOWER PAD TOE RAISE ON UNIVERSAL TYPE LEG PRESS MACHINE

Muscle Group: Main calf muscles
Degree of Difficulty: Intermediate

Sit on the back supported chair of a Universal type leg press machine. Hold on to the sides of the seat under your buttocks. Place the balls of your feet on the two lower pads provided and press the weight stack out until your legs are straight and your knees lock. Keep your legs in this position throughout the exercise. Inhale and press your feet forward as far as you comfortably can. Hold this position for a short period and then return your feet to the furthest back position you comfortably can and exhale. If you turn your toes out and heels in, it will affect the inner calf more. If you turn your feet straight, it will affect the main calf muscle more. If you turn your toes in and heels out, it will affect the outside of the calf more.

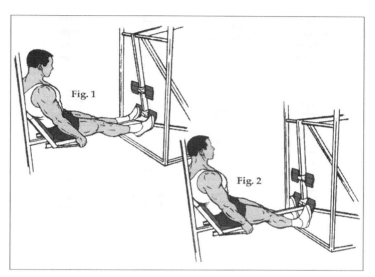

Sets/Reps: 3-4 sets of 20-25 reps

Date	Set One		Set Two		Set Three		Set Four	
	Reps	Weight	Reps	Weight	Reps	Weight	Reps	Weight

Muscle Group: Upper abdominals
Degree of Difficulty: Intermediate

Sit down on a sit-up board and hook your feet under the strap. With your knees bent to about a 45° angle, put your hands behind your head and place your chin on your chest. This will keep a slight bow to your back. From this position, inhale and lie back until your lower back touches the board. Exhale as you return to starting position.

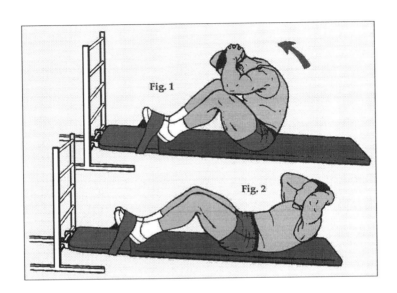

Sets/Reps: 1 set of 15-30 reps

	Set One					
Date	Reps	Weight				

INCLINE LEG PULL-IN

Muscle Group: Lower abdominals
Degree of Difficulty: Intermediate

Position a sit-up board on a 25-30° angle. Lie on the board with your head at the top Use your hands to hold yourself in a stationary position. Inhale and bend your knees while pulling your upper thighs into your midsection. Return to starting position and exhale. Concentrate on your lower abdominals during the exercise. Do not let your feet touch the board once you have started the exercise.

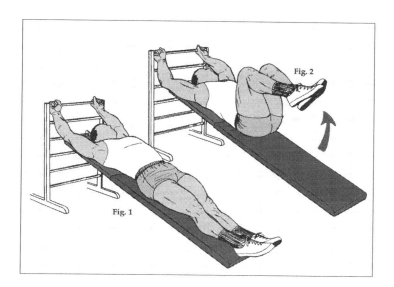

Fig. 2

Fig. 1

Sets/Reps: 1 set of 15-30 reps

	Set One					
Date	Reps	Weight				

Chapter 6

Month 5

Exercise	
1. Seated Barbell Twist	1 set of 25-50 reps
2. Flat Footed Medium Stance Barbell Nonlock Squat	3-5 sets of 8-10 reps
3. Standing Toe Raise on Hack Thrust Machine	3-5 sets of 20-25 reps
4. Medium Grip Barbell Bench Press	3-5 sets of 8-10 reps
5. Standing Palms In Dumbbell Press	3-5 sets of 8-10 reps
6. Bent Over Two Arm Long Bar Rowing	3-5 sets of 8-10 reps
7. Straight Arm Dumbbell Pullover	3-5 sets of 8-10 reps
8. Standing Dumbbell Triceps Curl	3-5 sets of 8-10 reps
9. Seated Concentrated Dumbbell Curl	3-5 sets of 8-10 reps
10. Jackknife Sit-Up	1 set of 10-30 reps

This is the next to last month of the beginner phase, and there's one big change: We've decreased the number of repetitions for most of the exercises you do eight to 10 reps, down from the 10 to 12 you have been doing. The lower reps enable you to handle more weight, which adds to the training intensity. This, in turn, gears you up for the intermediate phase.

I've also altered the sequence in which you work your body. During the previous two months, of course, you trained your body parts in this order: chest, back, deltoids, triceps, biceps, thighs, calves and midsection. This month the order is midsection, thighs, calves, chest, deltoids, back, triceps, biceps and midsection again. That will basically be the order you will use next month as well.

Here's a brief thumbnail sketch, so to speak, of where we're going.

You do a whole-body routine throughout the six months of the beginner phase and for the first four months of the six-month intermediate phase. In other words, you train your entire body in every workout for the first 10 months of the program.

The big change for the intermediate phase is that there are more exercises per workout. You generally perform 14 to 15 exercises per session compared to the nine or 10 you do during the beginner phase. The number of exercises per workout does not go much higher during the advanced phase, but you do more sets. In fact, the workload progression in this program increases from a range of 26 to 42 sets in the last two months of the beginner phase to ranges of 39 to 53 sets for the intermediate phase and 43 to 60 sets for most of the advanced phase.

Starting with the fifth month of the intermediate phase - or exactly halfway through the 20-month program—you make a significant switch from a whole-body routine to a split routine. From then on you train half of your body in one workout and the other half in the next. Also, instead of training three times a week, as you do during the first half of the program, you train six times a week - in order to continue to work each muscle group three times a week.

This change in the last two months of the intermediate phase is actually a way to get you revved up for the eight-month advanced phase. You continue using a split routine during most of the advanced phase, training six days a week; however, during the latter part of the advanced phase you switch to the approach most of the top pros use - working only two or three body parts per session.

Your task is to work hard enough to make consistent progress e route to your ultimate goal - what ever that is - but not overtrain, which will cause your enthusiast to wane and your progress to slot to a crawl.

Play It Safe

People who have low-back problems - and many have them - may experience some difficulty with an exercise like the barbell squat, which is included in this workout. If you have any low-back instability, I recommend that you do the following:

Use a weight that you are sure is not going to cause injury to or any excess strain on your lower back. If this weight is so light that it's not challenging to do eight to 10 squats per set, increase the repetitions rather than the weight and do 18, 20 or more reps to give the muscles involved a workout.

If you find that even a light weight aggravates your

back in a squat exercise, pick another thigh movement - such as leg presses or some other exercise that's done in a seated or supported position so that your low back is stable throughout. It's better to play it safe than to run the risk of injury, particularly since there are so many thigh movements to choose from.

Let me add, however, that if you adhere to strict form and you are conservative in the weight you use, you should be able to squat safely even if you have had back problems. You probably wouldn't think twice about doing an exercise such as standing calf raises - bad back or not - yet standing calf raises can be more threatening than squats to people who have low-back problems, especially if they try to use a lot of weight. When you stand erect on a calf raise machine with a lot of weight on your back, you are using your low back as if it were an automobile's universal joint. All that stress is on your back as you raise and lower the weight.

There's less trauma to your back when you do squats because your body adjusts to the biomechanics. The chief danger in the squat, of course, is that when you handle weights that feel heavy, you start to either round or arch your back - and when you do that, you put stress on the area and run the risk of blowing your back out.

In the final analysis, of course, you must use your own discretion. If you have a back problem, the rule of thumb is, Play it safe - and either use poundages on the squat that don't present a danger or choose thigh exercises on which you have some built-in stability or support for your back.

Another good idea is to do a good low-back warm-up or stretching movement before attempting any kind of squat exercise. In this routine the seated barbell twist serves that purpose for the barbell squat, which follows it.

Training Suggestions for Month 5

- For best results do this routine three times a week Monday, Wednesday and Friday or Tuesday, Thursday and Saturday Use the off days for rest and recuperation.
- Last month you progressed to four sets tar most of the movements. This month I suggest that on exercises 2 through 9 you use the following progression:
  - Week1: Three sets and minimum reps.
  - Week2: Four sets and medium reps.
  - Weeks 3 and 4: Five sets and maximum reps.
- For the two midsection exercises start out with the minimum number of reps and gradually increase the number so you're doing the upper end of the range

at the end of the month.
- Do not train to failure. The last rep should feel difficult but should not be an all-out effort. At the beginning of this routine you'll have to experiment to determine the poundages to use in order to make the last rep or two challenging but not impossible. Don't hesitate to decrease your weight on the last set or two of an exercise in order to complete the necessary number of reps. Finish what you start - don't train to failure.
- From week to week as your body adapts and your strength improves, increase the weight on each exercise. Remember, you want to make the last rep of each set challenging. Keep accurate records of your poundages, sets and reps from workout to workout. This will enable you to easily keep track of your progress from one poundage to the next rather than forcing you to rely on memory.
- Concentrate on correct form and mentally focus on the bodypart you're working.
- Rest for 30 seconds to two minutes between sets. If you feel any kind of unusual pain during your workout, consult with a trainer (if one is available). Of course, if you're just starting a training program, you should always check with a physician to ensure that you have no health problems that could make training dangerous.

SEATED BARBELL TWIST

Muscle Group: Obliques

Degree of Difficulty: Easy

Sit on the end of a bench with your feet planted firmly on the floor. Place a barbell on the back of your shoulders. Grasp the barbell with both hands in a comfortable position. Now, twist your torso to the right and then to the left by twisting at the waist only. Do not move your head from side to side as you perform this exercise. Be sure to keep your back straight and your head up. You inhale to the right and exhale to the left.

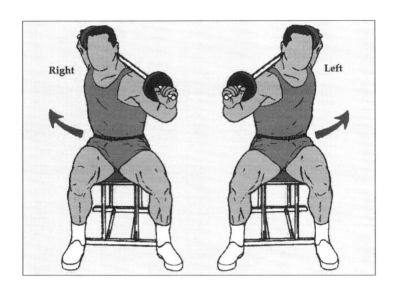

Sets/Reps: 1 set of 25-50 reps

	Set One					
Date	Reps	Weight				

FLAT FOOTED MEDIUM STANCE BARBELL NONLOCK SQUAT

Muscle Group: Upper thighs

Degree of Difficulty: Intermediate

Place a barbell on your upper back. Help stabilize the bar with a hand grip and spacing that feels most comfortable to you. Keep your head up, back straight, and your feet planted firmly on the floor about sixteen inches apart. Inhale and squat down until your upper thighs are parallel with the floor. Your head should remain up, back straight, and knees slightly to the sides. Return to starting position and exhale but do not lock your legs out or take a short rest before starting the next repetition. Immediately start the squat over again until the prescribed number of repetitions are completed.

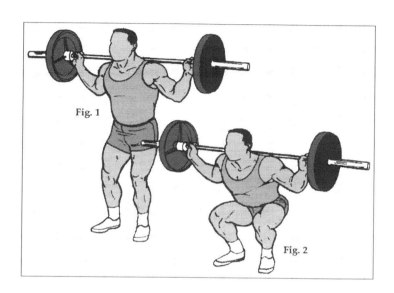

Fig. 1

Fig. 2

Sets/Reps: 3-5 sets of 8-10 reps

Date	Set One		Set Two		Set Three		Set Four		Set Five	
	Reps	Weight	Reps	Weight	Reps	Weight	Reps	Weight	Reps	Weight

Muscle Group: Main calf muscles

Degree of Difficulty: Intermediate

(The type of hack thrust machine you use will determine how you position yourself for this exercise. Regardless, the basic movement is the same.) Position your shoulders under the extended portion of a hack thrust machine or grasp the bars on each side of the sled with both hands keeping your arms straight. Stand on the slanted platform while facing into the machine. Stand erect with your back straight, head up and legs locked during the entire exercise. Do not let your hips move backward and forward while performing the exercise. Inhale and raise up on your toes as high as possible. Hold this position for a short period and return to starting position, dropping your heels as low as possible without having them touch the platform and exhale. If you turn your toes out and heels in, it will affect the inner calf more. If you keep your feet straight, it will affect the main calf muscle more. If you turn your toes in and heels out, it will affect the outside of the calf more.

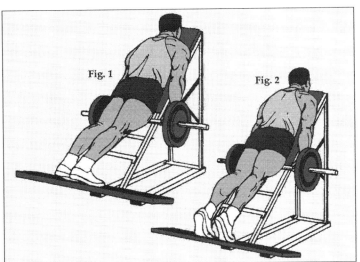

Sets/Reps: 3-5 sets of 20-25 reps

	Set One		Set Two		Set Three		Set Four		Set Five	
Date	Reps	Weight	Reps	Weight	Reps	Weight	Reps	Weight	Reps	Weight

MEDIUM GRIP BARBELL BENCH PRESS

Muscle Group: Outer pectorals

Degree of Difficulty: Intermediate

Lie in a supine position on a flat bench with your legs positioned at the sides of the bench and your feet flat on the floor. Using a hand grip that is about six inches wider than your shoulder width, bring the barbell to arm's length above the chest but in line with the shoulders. Lower the barbell to a position on the chest that is about an inch below the nipples of the pectorals. Note from figure 1 that the elbows are back and the chest is held high. Inhale as the barbell is lowered to the chest and exhale as you push the barbell back to arm's length. Do not relax and drop the weight on the chest but lower it with complete control making a definite pause at the chest before pressing it back to starting position. Keep the head on the bench and do not arch the back too sharply as to raise your hips off the bench.

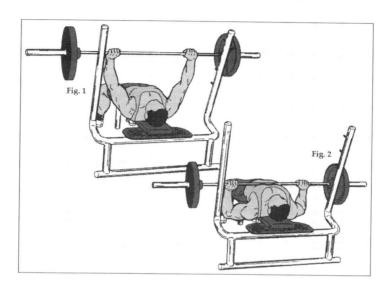

Sets/Reps: 3-5 sets of 8-10 reps

Date	Set One Reps	Weight	Set Two Reps	Weight	Set Three Reps	Weight	Set Four Reps	Weight	Set Five Reps	Weight

STANDING PALMS IN DUMBBELL PRESS

Muscle Group: Front and outer deltoids

Degree of Difficulty: Intermediate

Clean two dumbbells to shoulder height. Lock the legs and hips solidly. This will give you a solid platform from which to push. Keep the elbows in slightly and have the palms of the hands facing each other. Press the weights overhead to arm's length. Lower the weights to starting position, keeping the elbows in. Inhale before the press and exhale when lowering the dumbbells.

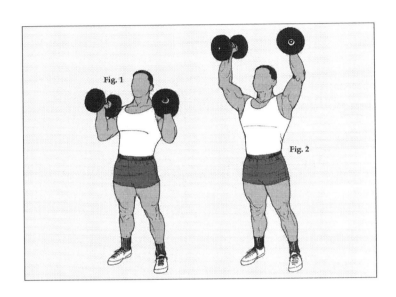

Sets/Reps: 3-5 sets of 8-10 reps

Date	Set One		Set Two		Set Three		Set Four		Set Five	
	Reps	Weight	Reps	Weight	Reps	Weight	Reps	Weight	Reps	Weight

BENT OVER TWO ARM LONG BAR ROWING

Muscle Group: Lats

Degree of Difficulty: Intermediate

Straddle a rowing bar with your feet about thirty-six inches apart. Bend down and grasp the bar with both hands. Keep your knees bent and your back straight but bent to about a 45° angle. Inhale and pull the bar up until the tops of your hands touch the lower part of your rib cage. Lower the bar to starting position and exhale. Do not let the weights touch the floor once you have begun the exercise. Keep the same fixed body position.

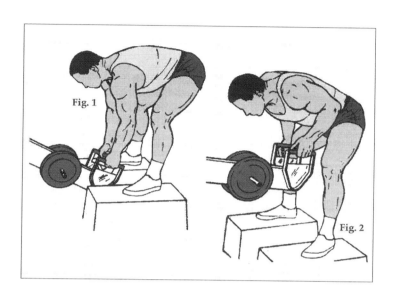

Sets/Reps: 3-5 sets of 8-10 reps

Date	Set One		Set Two		Set Three		Set Four		Set Five	
	Reps	Weight	Reps	Weight	Reps	Weight	Reps	Weight	Reps	Weight

Muscle Group: Pectorals and rib cage
Degree of Difficulty: Intermediate

Lie supine on a flat bench with your head as close to the end of the bench as possible. Place your hands flat against the inside plate of a dumbbell. With the dumbbell held at arm's length above the chest, take a deep breath and lower the dumbbell in a semicircular motion over the chest and head to a position behind your head that brings no discomfort to the shoulder area. From this position, return the dumbbell to starting position, still keeping the elbows in a locked position. Exhale as you reach the starting position. Keep the head down, your chest held high, breathe deeply and do not raise your hips off the bench.

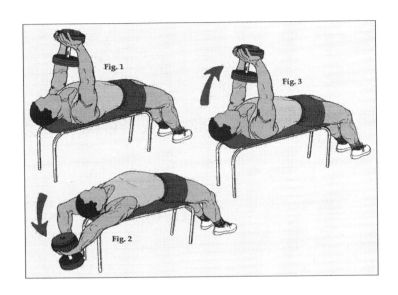

Sets/Reps: 3-5 sets of 8-10 reps

Date	Set One		Set Two		Set Three		Set Four		Set Five	
	Reps	Weight	Reps	Weight	Reps	Weight	Reps	Weight	Reps	Weight

STANDING DUMBBELL TRICEPS CURL

Muscle Group: Triceps
Degree of Difficulty: Difficult

Grasp one dumbbell with both hands and raise it overhead to arm's length, vertical with the floor. As you are raising the dumbbell rotate your hands up and over until the top plates are resting in the palms of your hands while your thumbs remain around the handle. Stand erect with your back straight, head up and feet about sixteen inches apart. Keep your upper arms in close to the sides of your head during the exercise. Inhale and lower the dumbbell behind your head in a semicircular motion until your forearms and biceps touch. Return the weight to starting position using a similar path and exhale.

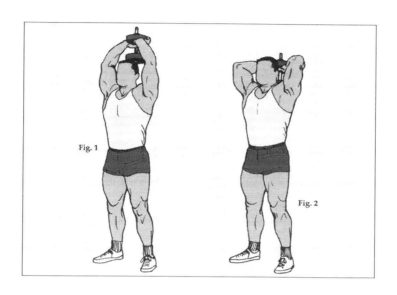

Sets/Reps: 3-5 sets of 8-10 reps

	Set One		Set Two		Set Three		Set Four		Set Five	
Date	Reps	Weight	Reps	Weight	Reps	Weight	Reps	Weight	Reps	Weight

Muscle Group: Biceps

Degree of Difficulty: Intermediate

Grasp a dumbbell in your right hand and sit on a bench with your feet about twenty-four inches apart. Position the dumbbell in front of you hanging at arm's length between your legs with a palms-up grip. Bend slightly at the waist and place your left hand on your left knee to help support your upper body. Rest your upper right arm against your inner right thigh about four inches above your knee. Inhale and curl the dumbbell upward in a semicircular motion by bending your arm at the elbow and keeping your upper arm vertical with the floor. Continue the curl until your biceps and forearm are touching. At the top position the dumbbell should be shoulder height. Return to starting position using a similar motion and exhale. Do the prescribed number of repetitions with your right arm and then change positions doing the same number of repetitions with your left arm.

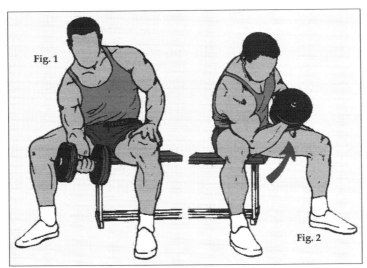

Sets/Reps: 3-5 sets of 8-10 reps

Date	Set One		Set Two		Set Three		Set Four		Set Five	
	Reps	Weight	Reps	Weight	Reps	Weight	Reps	Weight	Reps	Weight

JACKKNIFE SIT-UP

Muscle Group: Upper and lower abdominals

Degree of Difficulty: Difficult

Lie on the floor in a supine position. Place your arms behind your head at arms' length. You then bend at the waist while raising your legs and arms up at the same time, coming together vertically above your waist. Lower your arms and legs back to the floor to complete the repetition. Inhale as you commence the exercise and exhale as you finish. Keep your elbows and knees locked out during the exercise.

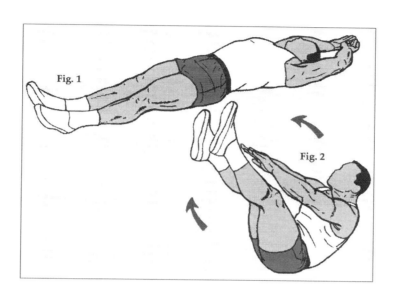

Sets/Reps: 1 set of 10-30 reps

	Set One				
Date	Reps	Weight			

Chapter 7

Month 6

Exercise	
1. Barbell Good Morning	1 set of 25-30 reps
2. Barbell Front Lunge	3-5 sets of 8-10 reps
3. Standing Toe Raise on Power Rack	3-5 sets of 20-25 reps
4. Inner Pec Press on Inner Pec Machine	3-5 sets of 8-10 reps
5. Medium Grip Barbell Upright Rowing	3-5 sets of 8-10 reps
6. Wide Grip Rear Lat Pull-Down	3-5 sets of 8-10 reps
7. Lying Supine Two Dumbbell Triceps Curl	3-5 sets of 8-10 reps
8. Standing Medium Grip Barbell Curl	3-5 sets of 8-10 reps
9. Over a Bench Sit-Up	1 set of 25-50 reps
10. Dip Stand Alternated Leg Raise	1 set of 25-50 reps

During this month, which concludes the beginner phase of the program, you train the various parts of your body in the same order as you did last month, following the same set-and-rep schemes - three to five sets for most of the exercises and eight to ten reps.

You may have noticed that I always recommend higher reps on the calf exercises - because 20 and 25. Experience has shown me that it's best to keep the repetitions high on calf work just as you have to do on forearm work - because the calf is a very dense muscle and seems to respond better to higher repetitions. Muscles like the biceps and triceps, on the other hand, are less dense, more coarse and respond better to lower reps. Consequently, my suggestion for calf exercises is to perform the same number of sets as you do for the other muscles but keep the reps much higher - doing 20 to 25 per set on all calf movements.

Note that the barbell front lunge, which is the second exercise in this program, calls for you to alternate legs, putting one foot forward, bringing it back, then putting the other foot forward and bringing it back. That's one rep. As you perform the exercise, you count the reps, "One, one; two, two; three, three" and so on until you get to the required number.

As for the number of sets, you have undoubtedly noticed as you have followed this training program that you generally drop back on the number of sets per exercise at the beginning of the month compared to what you were doing at the end of the previous month. That's the case again this time; at the end of last month you were doing five sets for most of the exercises, but at the beginning of this month I recommend that you go back to three sets per exercise and build back up.

Why? If you train with the proper intensity constantly increasing your poundages as you get stronger so that the last rep or two is always challenging but not an all-out, train-to-failure effort - you will find that at the end of the four weeks on any of these monthly routines you will have reached the maximum of your capability. you will be getting to the point where you are almost not going to be able to do the exercises properly - that is, in strict form - because the weight you are using is verging on the most that you can handle. That will mean you have reached a plateau in your strength progression for that exercise.

At that point of course, it becomes almost as difficult psychologically to do the workout as it is physiologically. Consequently, it only makes sense for you to back off psychologically at the beginning of the next month by decreasing the number of sets and then gradually build back up for another peak, as it were, in the last week or so of the cycle.

That's why the program usually calls for you to cut back on the number of sets per exercise at the beginning of each month.

The Choice Is Yours

This month's routine brings you to the end of the beginner phase of the program. Next month you move into the intermediate phase.

This seems like a good time to remind you that while this 20-month program gets progressively harder as we go from beginner to intermediate to advanced levels, the choice of how far you want to go or exactly what you want to do with these workouts is entirely up to you.

No doubt you have already noticed that you could become a very fit individual and look like a million bucks just by continuing to train at the present level - without ever going any further in terms of training workload or intensity. If you want to take your physique development above and beyond that - in other words, if you are truly dedicated to perfecting your physique and you have the time, energy and drive to do it - then the intermediate and advanced programs will help you get there.

If you do want to back off at some point and just carry on with the previous month's training intensity, remember that you can maintain what you have built - and remain an extremely fit, muscle-toned individual - simply by changing the exercises each month and continuing with the same number of sets and reps you have been doing. You can also use the routines from the intermediate and advanced phases but keep the sets and reps at the beginner level; i.e., three to five sets, eight to 10 or 10 to 12 reps.

You can play all kinds of creative games with these monthly routines. In fact, that may be necessary because some people may need more time than others to work up to the more advanced levels of training.

So as we go on with this program, you have all kinds of options open to you - which is the whole idea because it's your life and your body. Only you know how much time and energy you can devote to your training, how far you want to go with it and ultimately what you want to achieve, so it's only right that you be the one to call the shots.

I am just here to give you the exercises and some guidance on how to accomplish what it is you want to accomplish. First and last, however, the choice of what you want to accomplish is yours, which is as it should be. To shine own self be true.

Training Suggestions for Month 6

- For best results do this routine three times a week - Monday, Wednesday and Friday or Tuesday, Thursday and Saturday. Use the off days for rest and recuperation.
- Last month you worked up to five sets for most of the exercises. This month I suggest that on exercises 2 through 8 you drop back to three set initially and then follow this progression through the month:
  - Week1: Three sets and minimum reps.
  - Week2: Four sets and medium reps.
  - Weeks 3 and 4: Five sets and maximum reps.
- For the three midsection exercises in this routine start with the minimum number of repetitions and grad-

ually increase them so you do the maximum number at the end of the month.

- Do not train to failure. The last rep should feel difficult but should not be an all-out effort. At the beginning of this routine you'll have to experiment to determine the poundages to use in order to make the last rep or two challenging but not impossible. Don't hesitate to decrease your weight on the last set or two of an exercise in order to complete the necessary number of reps. Finish what you start - don't train to failure.
- From week to week as your body adapts and your strength improves, increase the weight on each exercise. Remember, you want to make the last rep of each set challenging. Keep accurate records of your poundages, sets and reps from workout to workout. This will enable you to easily keep track of your progress from one poundage to the next rather than forcing you to rely on memory.
- Concentrate on correct form and mentally focus on the bodypart you're working.
- Rest for 30 seconds to two minutes between sets. If you feel any kind of unusual pain during your workout, consult with a trainer (if one is available). Of course, if you're just starting a training program, you should always check with a physician to ensure that you have no health problems that could make training dangerous.

BARBELL GOOD MORNING

Muscle Group: Lower back and abdominals
Degree of Difficulty: Easy

Stand erect with your feet about sixteen inches apart. Place a light barbell on your shoulders. Grasp the bar with both hands in a comfortable position. Keep your back straight and your head up as you inhale and bend forward at the waist until your upper body is parallel to the floor. Return to starting position and exhale. Be sure your knees are in a locked position during the entire exercise.

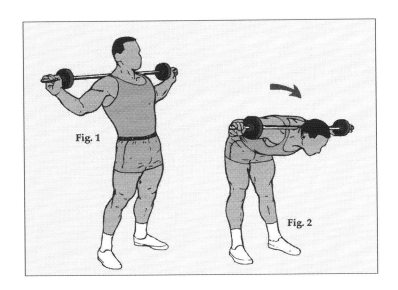

Fig. 1

Fig. 2

Sets/Reps: 1 set of 25-30 reps

	Set One					
Date	Reps	Weight				

BARBELL FRONT LUNGE

Muscle Group: Thighs and thigh biceps
Degree of Difficulty: Difficult

Place a barbell on your rear shoulders as if you were to perform a barbell squat. Keep your head up, back straight and feet planted firmly on the floor about fourteen inches apart. Inhale and step forward as far as possible with your right leg until your upper right thigh is almost parallel with the floor. Your left leg should be held as straight as possible, not bending the knee any more than is necessary. From this position, step back to starting position and exhale. Do the prescribed number of repetitions with your right leg and then repeat the same number of repetitions with your left leg.

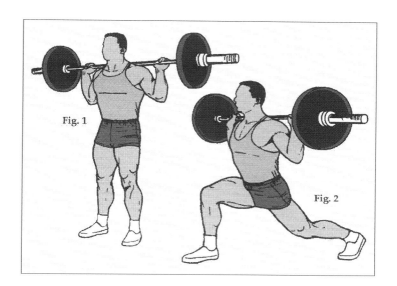

Fig. 1

Fig. 2

Sets/Reps: 3-5 sets of 8-10 reps

Date	Set One		Set Two		Set Three		Set Four		Set Five	
	Reps	Weight	Reps	Weight	Reps	Weight	Reps	Weight	Reps	Weight

Muscle Group: Main calf muscles
Degree of Difficulty: Intermediate

Place a barbell on the pegs of a power rack just below shoulder height. Position a thick board, or raised platform, directly under the barbell. Place the barbell on your upper back keeping the bar against the power rack throughout the exercise. Stand erect with your back straight, head up and legs straight with your knees locked as you stand with the balls of your feet on the board. Do not let your hips move backward or forward while performing the exercise. Inhale and raise up on your toes as high as possible. Hold this position a short period and return to starting position and exhale. Be sure to keep the bar against the rack. If you turn your toes out and heels in, it will affect your inner calf more. If you keep your feet straight, it will affect your main calf muscle more. If you turn your toes in and heels out, it will affect the outside of your calf more.

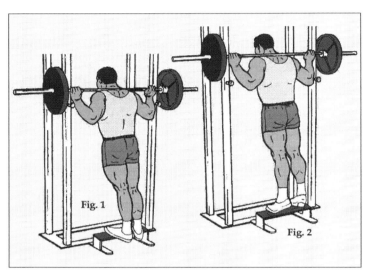

Fig. 1   Fig. 2

Sets/Reps: 3-5 sets of 20-25 reps

Date	Set One		Set Two		Set Three		Set Four		Set Five	
	Reps	Weight	Reps	Weight	Reps	Weight	Reps	Weight	Reps	Weight

INNER PEC PRESS ON INNER PEC MACHINE

Muscle Group: Upper and inner pectorals
Degree of Difficulty: Intermediate

The way this exercise is performed will depend a great deal on how the inner pec machine you use is constructed. Some are more elaborate than others and have adjustable seats and arms. The main thing is to remember while performing this exercise is to keep the upper arms fairly high and about in line with your shoulders. You should keep the forearms in a vertical position so as not to bring any more of the triceps and deltoids into play than necessary. Concentrate on squeezing your forearms together by concentrating on the pectorals doing the work. Inhale as you are squeezing and exhale as you return your arms back to starting position.

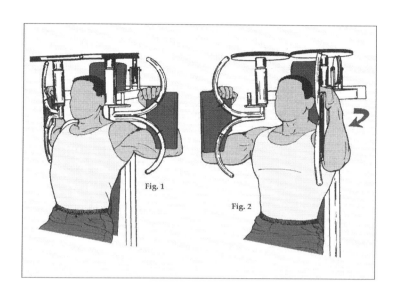

Fig. 1   Fig. 2

Sets/Reps: 3-5 sets of 8-10 reps

	Set One		Set Two		Set Three		Set Four		Set Five	
Date	Reps	Weight	Reps	Weight	Reps	Weight	Reps	Weight	Reps	Weight

Muscle Group: Front deltoids and trapezius
Degree of Difficulty: Intermediate

Place your hands on a barbell with the palms facing down and use a hand grip about eighteen inches apart. With the barbell at arm's length while you are standing erect and in a stationary position, pull the weight straight up until it is nearly under the chin. Keep the elbows out to the sides and in the top position the elbows are nearly as high as your ears. Keep the barbell in close to the body and pause momentarily at the top before letting the weight back to starting position. Inhale as you raise the bar and exhale as you lower the bar.

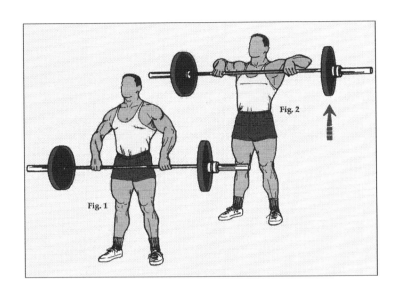

Sets/Reps: 3-5 sets of 8-10 reps

	Set One		Set Two		Set Three		Set Four		Set Five	
Date	Reps	Weight	Reps	Weight	Reps	Weight	Reps	Weight	Reps	Weight

WIDE GRIP REAR LAT PULL-DOWN

Muscle Group: Upper lats
Degree of Difficulty: Intermediate

Place your hand on a lat machine bar about thirty-six inches apart. Kneel down on your knees until you are supporting the weight stack with your arms while they are extended overhead. Inhale and pull the bar down behind your head to the middle of your neck. Return to starting position ant exhale. Keep your back straight and do no bend forward.

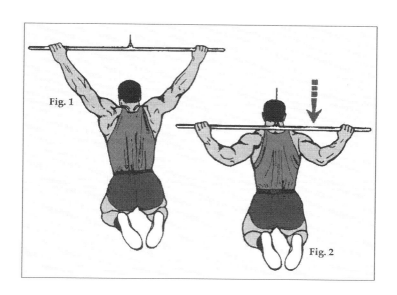

Sets/Reps: 3-5 sets of 8-10 reps

Date	Set One		Set Two		Set Three		Set Four		Set Five	
	Reps	Weight	Reps	Weight	Reps	Weight	Reps	Weight	Reps	Weight

Muscle Group: Triceps
Degree of Difficulty: Intermediate

Lie on a flat bench. Hold a dumbbell in each hand and press them to arm's length keeping them in line with your shoulders. Inhale and lower both dumbbells straight down in a semicircular motion by bending your arms at the elbows but keeping your upper arms vertical throughout the exercise. The dumbbells should be lowered until your forearms and biceps touch. Press the dumbbells back to starting position using the same path and exhale.

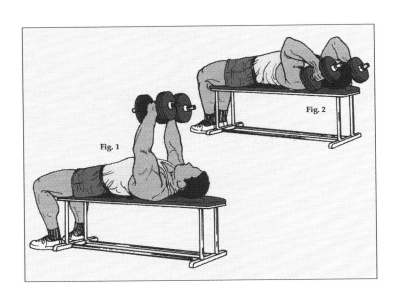

Sets/Reps: 3-5 sets of 8-10 reps

	Set One		Set Two		Set Three		Set Four		Set Five	
Date	Reps	Weight	Reps	Weight	Reps	Weight	Reps	Weight	Reps	Weight

STANDING MEDIUM GRIP BARBELL CURL

Muscle Group: Biceps

Degree of Difficulty: Intermediate

Hold a barbell with both hands using a palms-up grip about eighteen inches apart. Stand erect with your feet about sixteen inches apart. With the barbell at arm's length against your upper thighs, inhale and curl the bar up to the height of your shoulders keeping your back straight, legs and hips locked out. As you are lowering the bar back to starting position, do so in a controlled manner causing the biceps to resist the weight as much as possible. Exhale as you return to starting position.

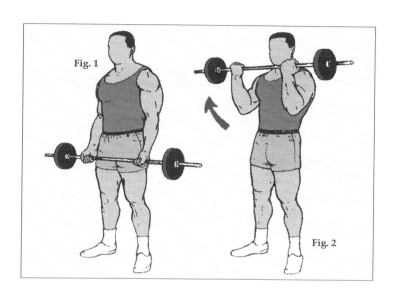

Sets/Reps: 3-5 sets of 8-10 reps

Date	Set One		Set Two		Set Three		Set Four		Set Five	
	Reps	Weight	Reps	Weight	Reps	Weight	Reps	Weight	Reps	Weight

Muscle Group: Upper abdominals
Degree of Difficulty: Intermediate

Position a bench so you are able to sit on it and have an object close by so you can put your feet under it to support your weight. Sit directly on the bench and your knees should have a slight bend to them. Starting at the upright position, inhale and lower your torso backwards and down until you are just below parallel with the floor. Return to starting position and exhale.

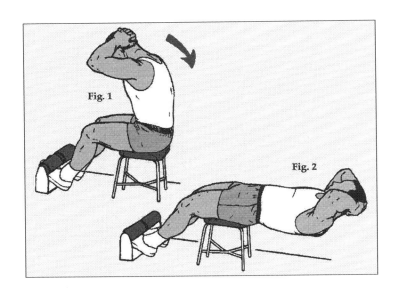

Sets/Reps: 1 set of 25-50 reps

	Set One				
Date	Reps	Weight			

DIP STAND ALTERNATED LEG RAISE

Muscle Group: Lower abdominals

Degree of Difficulty: Difficult

Position yourself on a dip stand facing away from the machine with your body being supported by your arms, having your elbows locked out. Hanging in a vertical position, inhale and raise your right leg up until it is parallel to the floor. As you commence to lower your right leg, start raising your left leg to give you the same motion your legs move while swimming. Inhale as you raise your right leg and exhale as you raise your left leg.

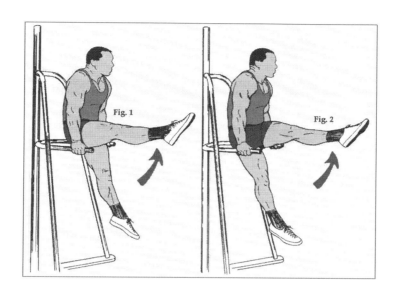

Sets/Reps: 1 set of 25-50 reps

	Set One					
Date	Reps	Weight				

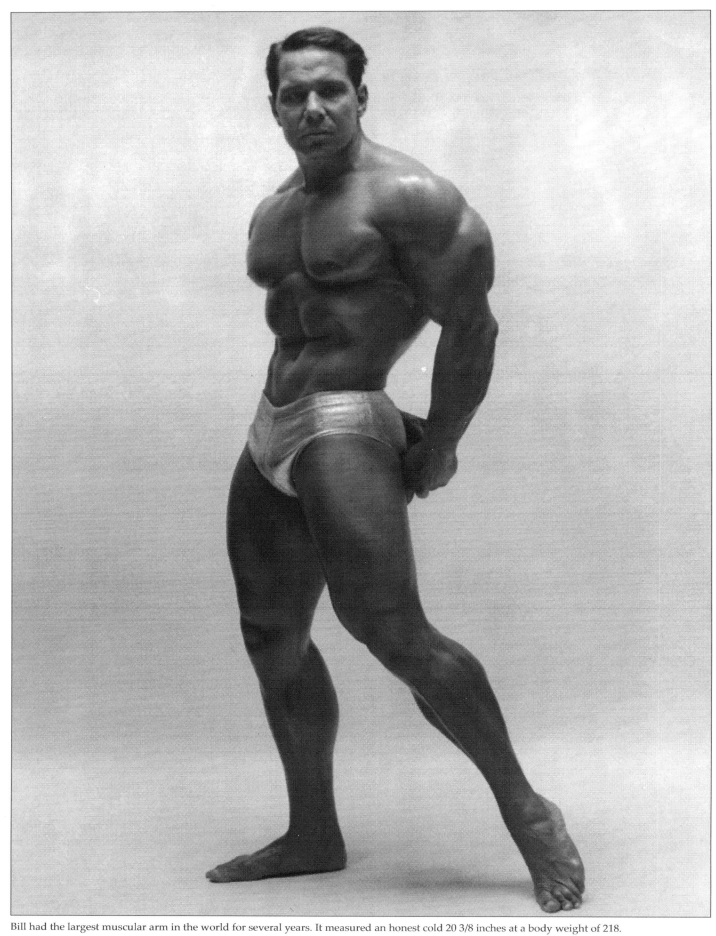

Bill had the largest muscular arm in the world for several years. It measured an honest cold 20 3/8 inches at a body weight of 218.

Made in the USA
San Bernardino, CA
26 October 2015